EPILEPSY

EPILEPSY

Allen H. Middleton, Ph.D.
Arthur A. Attwell, Ed.D.
and Gregory O. Walsh, M.D.

Little, Brown and Company   Boston–Toronto

First Edition

Drawing on page 4 adapted from an illustration by Anthony Ravielli from *The Human Brain* by Isaac Asimov. Copyright © 1963 by Isaac Asimov. Reprinted by arrangement with The New American Library, Inc., New York, New York.
Drawings on pages 5 and 6 adapted from illustrations in *Human Neuroanatomy* by Raymond C. Truex and Malcolm B. Carpenter. Copyright © 1969 by The Williams & Wilkins Company.

LIBRARY OF CONGRESS CATALOGING IN PUBLICATION DATA
Middleton, Allen H.
　　Epilepsy.
　　Bibliography: p. 226
　　Includes index.
　　1. Epilepsy. I. Attwell, Arthur A., and Walsh, Gregory, joint authors. II. Title [DNLM: 1. Epilepsy—Popular works. WL385 M628e]
　　RC372.M39　　　616.8′53　　　80–14192
　　ISBN 0–316–56952–6　　　AACR2

BP
Designed by Susan Windheim

Published simultaneously in Canada
by Little, Brown & Company (Canada) Limited
PRINTED IN THE UNITED STATES OF AMERICA

To Rita, Dottie, and Leita
and
to Richard B. and his family

CONTENTS

FOREWORD

Since historical times, the appearance of epilepsy in an individual has been viewed with fear, anxiety, and often despair. Owing to lack of knowledge regarding the origin and treatment of seizure disorders, afflicted persons became progressively more handicapped from the effects of uncontrolled convulsions, after being imprisoned, isolated in institutions, or hidden away at home.

Understandably, parents and epileptic individuals themselves considered the presence of this condition a hopeless situation that would ultimately result in severe mental and physical damage precluding any chance of a normal life.

With the advent in the past forty to fifty years of new diagnostic methods and development of effective medications for seizure control, prospects for the person with epilepsy have radically changed. Unfortunately, the general public and many professionals and paraprofessionals are not aware of these changes. To bridge this gap, the authors of *Epilepsy* have brought together in clear, concise, question-and-answer format a remarkable synthesis of knowledge in the field of epilepsy.

Parents of children having epilepsy will find this book invaluable. The authors are particularly skilled in enumerating and answering the many questions and anxieties faced by the parent and the individual with epilepsy. Being aware that the parental attitude evoked by epilepsy, especially in the very early stages, is significant in determining the child's life adjustment, the authors have sensitively reviewed important social and personal factors that may condition the response of the parent. This book should be in the hands of all parents with an epileptic child.

For medical, psychology, and nursing students as well as professionals already practicing, the review of the diagnosis, treatment, and classifications of epilepsy contains material not seen in conventional textbooks. All those in professional disciplines as well as parents will greatly appreciate the comprehensive review of service referral sources and training aids available in the field of epilepsy. There are also extensive reading lists for the parent, student, or professional seeking more detailed study.

Lastly, the authors are to be commended not only for the skills and experience they have infused into their writing but also for hours of dedicated reading and research that resulted in this excellent compendium on epilepsy.

Mary Lu Hickman, M.D.
Medical Director
Central Valley Regional Center
Fresno, California

INTRODUCTION

One of our most baffling disorders, and perhaps still the one most shrouded with misconception, is epilepsy. It has plagued us for centuries and affects an estimated three to four million Americans today. As a neurological disorder, it is second only to mental retardation. Even as short a time as a generation ago, almost any type of seizure was referred to as "the fits," and employers and educators alike showed a reluctance to accept those afflicted. It is hard to imagine that at one time certain states in our own country even refused to issue a marriage license to anyone with epilepsy!

Thankfully, science and research have gradually replaced prejudice and misunderstanding with public enlightenment. Medicine has further dissolved the veil of mystery with its almost unbelievable advancement in containing most types of seizures. Organizations such as the Epilepsy Foundation of America have kept the public informed and have provided public access to brochures, facilities, legal information, and the like. Schools are learning that the child with seizures can be considered a normal pupil in every way, and most employers have already learned that the person *with epilepsy* is no greater risk than the one *without epilepsy* in appropriate jobs.

This book is still another attempt to bring epilepsy even farther "out of the shadows." It has been written in lay language for the parent as well as the professional, who is often confronted with questions about seizure disorders and their management. The questions in this book are typical of those which have been asked of the authors and others through the years by patients and parents of children with epilepsy.

The authors recognize that raising a child with epilepsy requires greater knowledge and understanding on the part of the parents than raising children who are not handicapped. We hope this book will be of value to families in the process of meeting this challenge.

It is important for everyone to recognize that with proper treatment and a supportive family, individuals with epilepsy can lead active and normal lives.

The authors gratefully acknowledge the cooperation of the Epilepsy Foundation of America in supplying information and literature, which have been cited throughout the book, and for reviewing the manuscript. Individuals we would like to thank are Pamela McGarvey, Susan Ames, Peter Van Haverbeke, Sandy Kotschmaryk, Don Pogoloff, Sarah Fader, William Palmer, William Flynn, and Elhamy Khalil, M.D. A special measure of gratitude is extended to Mary Lu Hickman, M.D., for her suggestions in the early drafts of the text. A note of appreciation goes to Dr. Doris Fraser, Massachusetts Administrative Agency for the Developmentally Disabled. Our thanks also to Rita Middleton for editing, and to Betsy Pitha for copyediting, the text; and to Anna Barbour and Donna Love for the final preparation of the manuscript.

AHM, AAA, GOW
Visalia, California
June 1981

EPILEPSY

WHAT IS EPILEPSY?

What actually is epilepsy?

Epilepsy is not a disease in and of itself — it is a symptom of disease. Epilepsy is a condition in which a person has recurrent *seizures,* changes in behavior or activity brought on by an excessive electrical discharge in the brain cells. A seizure can be caused by *any* disease or accident that affects the central nervous system.

The seizures in epilepsy are sudden, episodic, and recurrent. The varieties of seizures are almost infinite because any area of the brain can be affected by the abnormal electrical discharge. Seizures can range from a total lapse of consciousness with stiffening and jerking of the whole body to just a staring off into space with a lapse of consciousness that lasts only a few seconds. Or the seizure may consist of just a single twitch of some body part, such as the face or hand or foot. Some seizure discharges take place in only a small part of the brain involved with some central nervous system function, such as memory or vision. Then the person may experience only a certain vivid memory or a feeling that things seem very familiar, or may seem to see flashing lights.

A single, isolated seizure resulting from some major stress on the body, such as infection, deprivation of sleep, abrupt withdrawal from alcohol or other drugs, or very high fever, is not necessarily considered epileptic. Seizures occurring in infants as a result of high fever are surprisingly frequent and by some estimates affect approximately 5 percent of the population. They may never happen again and do not mean the child will have epilepsy or recurrent seizures.

We are all potential seizure patients if our brains are stressed enough. Fortunately for most of us, the stress we undergo every day is not enough to cause abnormal electrical discharges in our brains, and so we do not have seizures. But in certain susceptible individuals, stress may precipitate seizures. If they continue, then that condition is called *epilepsy*, a chronic problem of recurrent seizures that may be of many different types depending upon the area of the brain involved in the seizure discharge and the duration of the discharge.

Is "epilepsy" the same as a "seizure disorder"?

The terms *epilepsy* and *seizure disorder* mean the same thing. Some people also use the word *convulsion* as equivalent to *seizure* and *epilepsy*, but if it is used at all, *convulsion* should refer only to the motor actions, or convulsive movements (jerks of the body), that are associated with certain types of seizures. There are seizures, as we shall see, in which no actual convulsion occurs.

Epilepsy comes from the Greek word *epilambanein*, which means "to seize" — hence, seizure disorder. Some people speak of *episodes*, *fits*, *attacks*, or *spells*. We prefer to use the term *seizure disorder* or *epilepsy*.

Is epilepsy a recently discovered condition, or has it been known for a long time?

Although epilepsy may seem to be a recent phenomenon, that is probably because of the publicity it has been receiving during the past few years. Actually, epilepsy has been observed as far back as history records. Symptoms known to be epileptic were observed in the ancient world; people then often felt that sufferers from epilepsy were possessed by supernatural beings or were divinely inspired. The disorder was sometimes called "the sacred illness." Around 400 B.C. the Greek physician Hippocrates made frequent mention of the condition in his writings. Though he was in error in believing epilepsy to be based on an imbalance of the four "humours" (blood, phlegm, yellow bile, and black bile), he did consider that the malfunction was involved with the brain.

Hippocrates was the first, and unfortunately the last for several centuries, to hold that epilepsy was a natural phenomenon arising within the body. During the Middle Ages, people continued to believe that seizures were of divine origin or were caused by demons or were always inherited or were contagious. Sufferers from epilepsy were kept isolated in hospitals, so that their breath would not contaminate others.

The list of famous historical people as well as modern-day personalities with this disorder is almost endless. Some of the historical figures believed to have had epilepsy were Alexander the Great, Caesar (his was called the "falling sickness"), Buddha, Napoleon, Handel, van Gogh (the painter's seizures were diagnosed as "non-focal symptomatic epilepsy, induced by consuming absinthe"), Dante, and Socrates. More recently, Tchaikovsky and Alfred Nobel are known to have had epilepsy. Some have conjectured that the Apostle Paul had epilepsy, though the evidence for this is rather scanty, based on his three-day blindness while on the road to Damascus, and his frequent mention of his "infirmity" and his "thorn in the side."

There are several successful and well-known actors and actresses who are able to maintain their time schedules and to be before the public with the knowledge that they might have a seizure at any time. One actress had a major seizure on a TV talk show, and returned later during the show to discuss the condition.

I don't know very much about the brain. Can you explain a little more?

Look at figure 1. The brain is divided into two halves, or *hemispheres*. Figure 1 shows a lateral (side) view of one hemisphere. Each hemisphere is divided into four areas, or *lobes:* the frontal lobe, the parietal lobe, the occipital lobe, and the temporal lobe. The groove that separates the frontal lobe from the parietal lobe is called the *central sulcus,* and the fissure that separates the temporal lobe from the frontal lobe is called the *lateral sulcus.* All the lobes have very complex functions. For simplification, these are the major ones: The frontal lobe is responsible for complex associations and body movements. The parietal lobe is responsible for fine sensations, such as being able to feel the difference between, say, cloth, wood, or metal with the hand. The occipital lobe is responsible for vision. The temporal lobe is responsible for the complexities of emotions, reactions to emotions, memory, smell, and hearing. The outer layer of the brain (the gray matter), in which most of these activities and events take place, is called the *cortex,* and the ridges between the fissures, or *sulci,* on the surface of the cortex are called *gyri.*

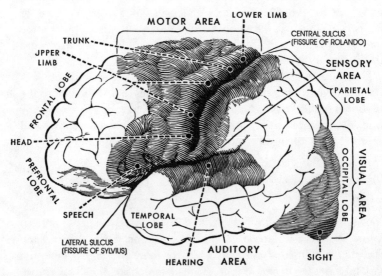

Fig. 1. Location of important areas of the cerebrum

The various motor areas of the body have matching areas in the frontal and parietal lobes of the brain. For example, the face and hands have very large areas of representation because many fine and subtle movements take place in these parts of the body. Conversely, the legs and chest have smaller areas of representation because their movements are much less fine. Figure 2 shows the various body parts in the motor areas of the brain, and figure 3 shows parts of the body drawn in proportion to the amount of the cortex they represent.

In general, the left hemisphere of the brain is responsible for movement of the right side of the body, and the right hemisphere governs movement of the left side of the body. Therefore, if a seizure

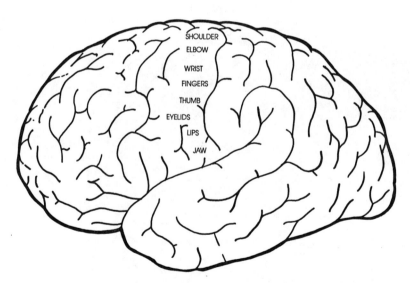

Fig. 2. Representation of parts of the body in the motor area on the surface of the brain

discharge starts on the left side of the brain in the motor area of the cortex responsible for the hand, the seizure manifestation will be a movement of the right hand. As the discharge spreads over the motor area in the brain, so the movement in the body will spread from the right hand to the arm, to the face, to the right side of the chest, to the right leg. The seizure discharge can start in the sensory area of the brain, which would mean that the seizure would manifest itself as a sensation down the opposite side of the body. The discharge, of course, can spread from the sensory to the motor cortex so that the seizure would start as a sensation and then become a movement; or the discharge could start in the motor cortex and then spread to the sensory cortex and become more of a sensation.

In the same way, if the seizure discharge starts in the occipital lobe of the brain, the patient may "see" some visual phenomena such as flashing lights or a bright light or lines (or any type of visual

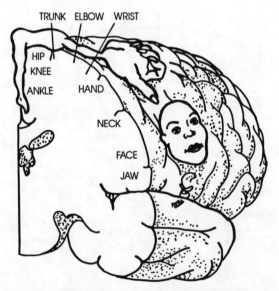

Fig. 3. Exaggeration of body parts in the motor cortex (a motor "homunculus"), drawn so that the sizes of the body parts are proportional to the sizes of the areas of cortical representation

pattern), depending on the discharge in the area involved. If the discharge is in the right visual cortex, the patient, because of the structure of the brain, will "see" the phenomena off to the left side of the body.

The brain is made up of several billion nerve cells *(neurons)* that are interconnected in extremely complicated arrangements. Neurons are so constructed that they generate and transmit tiny electrical impulses at very high speeds. The discharge of these impulses normally occurs in regular and orderly patterns. These patterns are called *brain waves,* and they can be recorded on the *electroencephalogram.* Through animal experimentation as well as observations of seizure patients a great deal has been learned about the electrical events that happen during a seizure and in between seizures, but the precise cause of that electrical event has not been exactly determined.

In animals the hallmark of a *seizure focus* (the particular location in the brain of the abnormal electric discharge) is a brain-wave pattern called a *spike-and-slow-wave discharge.* The spike phase shows an abnormally excitatory electrical output inside single brain cells; the slow-wave phase indicates an electrical input into the same cells that is inhibitory. Both phases are probably the result of thousands of neurons firing off simultaneously. The pattern occurs in its entirety only when there is no seizure. During a seizure the slow-wave phase disappears and only the spike phase occurs. It is probably the loss of the slow-wave inhibition that permits the excitatory output to get out of hand and cause the seizure.

A great deal of research has been devoted to just why all this takes place. Most likely it has something to do with the cell membrane and the sodium-potassium pump that is responsible for energy of that membrane. In addition, it may well have something to do with the biochemistry and neurophysiology of not only the brain cells themselves but also the supportive elements of the brain, called *glia.*

You have said that there are many varieties of seizures. What are they, and how do they differ?

Physicians who deal with epilepsy prefer to use the International Classification of Epileptic Seizures, which is given in the accompa-

INTERNATIONAL CLASSIFICATION OF EPILEPTIC SEIZURES

I. *Partial seizures* (seizures beginning locally)
   A.   *Partial seizures with elementary symptomatology (generally without impairment of consciousness)*
      1. With motor symptoms *[includes Jacksonian seizures]*
      2. With special sensory or somatosensory symptoms
      3. With autonomic symptoms
      4. Compound forms
   B.   *Partial seizures with complex symptomatology (generally with impairment of consciousness)*
      [temporal lobe or psychomotor seizures]
      1. With impairment of consciousness only
      2. With cognitive symptomatology
      3. With affective symptomatology
      4. With "psychosensory" symptomatology
      5. With "psychomotor" symptomatology (automatisms)
      6. Compound forms
   C.   *Partial seizures secondarily generalized*
II. *Generalized seizures* (bilaterally symmetrical and without local onset)
      1. Absences *[petit mal]*
      2. Bilateral massive epileptic myoclonus
      3. Infantile spasms
      4. Clonic seizures
      5. Tonic seizures
      6. Tonic-clonic seizures *[grand mal]*
      7. Atonic seizures
      8. Akinetic seizures
III. *Unilateral seizures* (or predominantly)
IV. *Unclassified epileptic seizures* (due to incomplete data)

Abstracted from H. Gastaut, "Clinical and electroencephalographical classification of epileptic seizures," *Epilepsia* 11 (1970): 102–113. The older terms for types of seizures are given in square brackets.

nying chart. The chart shows both the internationally agreed-upon terms for seizure types and the older terms, which are given in brackets.

In this classification, seizures basically are broken up into those that have a *partial*, or *focal, onset* in one single area of the brain and those that have a *generalized onset*. This concept is very important in understanding seizures and their treatment. Focal onset means that the abnormal electrical discharge starts in one certain area of the brain; the clinical manifestation, or change in behavior, brought about by the discharge depends upon the specific area of the brain involved at any particular point in time. As we've indicated, if the visual cortex of the brain is involved, the patient may see flashing lights or circles as the discharge moves over that area of the brain. If the seizure discharge involves the motor cortex, the clinical change may be either a single jerk or multiple jerks of the arm or leg or face. A Jacksonian seizure is one in which jerking in one area of the body — for instance, the hand — may then spread out over the rest of the arm and then to the face and leg, if the electrical discharge spreads out to involve that brain area. If the seizure discharge involves the sensory cortex of the brain, the patient may experience just a funny feeling or numbness or tingling over one side of the body. If the discharge involves the memory area of the brain, the patient may vividly recollect something seen or heard in the past. Partial seizures of this type do not affect or spread to areas of the brain involved with consciousness.

The second subcategory of focal-onset seizures ("partial seizures with complex symptomatology"; often called "partial complex" or "psychomotor" seizures) describes abnormal discharges that usually occur in both temporal lobes. These areas govern, as we have seen, memory and alertness. In these seizures, the patient generally experiences an impairment of consciousness, may undergo changes in thinking or memory ("cognitive" symptomatology), or in emotions ("affective" symptomatology), and may perform simple automatic actions ("psychomotor" symptomatology), such as walking, smacking the lips, picking at clothing, rubbing the hands, or opening a door. Usually the patient has no recall of the events occurring during the actual seizure, which may last for one or two minutes. It is important to remember that if the discharge involves both temporal lobes, particularly deep areas therein, the person will lose consciousness, although the eyes may be open and the automatic behavior mentioned above may continue. After the seizure the person may be confused.

The third, very important subcategory is "partial seizures secondarily generalized." Any seizure discharge beginning in one focal area of the brain, for instance, the temporal lobe, can start as a feeling of déjà vu (a feeling of familiarity) and then change into a partial complex seizure with a lapse or impairment of consciousness and with some automatic movement or behavior. Then, if the seizure discharge spreads out to the rest of the brain, the person can have a *secondarily generalized tonic-clonic (grand-mal)* seizure. It is something like a chain reaction: the abnormal discharge in a few brain cells kicks off abnormal discharges in more and more brain cells until the whole brain is involved. Very often it is this secondarily generalized tonic-clonic seizure that brings a person to the attention of a physician.

The second major class of seizures is "generalized onset seizures." These begin without a pinpointed, focal onset and affect both sides of the body (they are "bilaterally symmetrical"). In this category we find the two classic types of epilepsy most people think of: *absence,* or *petit-mal,* seizures; and *generalized tonic-clonic,* or *grand-mal,* seizures.

In the absence seizure, the patient stares straight ahead, is out of contact with the environment for a brief period (5 to 15 seconds), and may occasionally make a minor movement, like blinking the eyes. These seizures are often described as staring spells. After the episode, the person probably will immediately resume what he or she was doing and may or may not be aware of the brief interruption in normal activity. The seizures may occur dozens of times during the day. Petit mal is associated with a very characteristic pattern on the electroencephalogram, which we'll discuss in more detail below. What is important to remember here is that petit mal is a distinct disorder, not just a vague term for any seizure other than grand mal. Petit-mal seizures require treatment entirely different from that for other types of seizures and must be correctly identified.

Grand mal is more appropriately called generalized tonic-clonic seizures. *Tonic* refers to a stiffening of the body, and *clonic* refers to a jerking of the body. The patient usually stiffens for 30 to 60 seconds and then jerks for a like period; or the stiffening and jerking may alternate irregularly. The patient will lose consciousness and fall. Respiration is jerky and may be briefly suspended, the face becomes pale and then cyanotic, and the eyes may roll. There may be tongue-biting, urinary incontinence, and drooling. The seizures last from one to five minutes, after which the person may be confused and complain of fatigue or headache. Some individuals are drowsy and sleep after the seizure. Although generally there is awareness that a seizure has occurred, the individual does not remember what happened during the episode. The jerking muscle movements in grand mal are what is usually called a convulsion. (The seizure can also be pure tonic — stiffening — or pure clonic — jerking.)

"Bilateral massive epileptic myoclonus" and "infantile spasms" refer to sudden jerks of the whole body appearing in infants.

"Atonic" seizures are sometimes called "drop attacks": the patient will suddenly lose muscle tone, drop to the ground, and then just as suddenly get right back up and go about his or her business. It is difficult to determine whether there is any actual loss of consciousness in these attacks because they are so rapid and so short that it is hard to administer any tests.

An "akinetic" seizure is one in which there is simply a loss of movement. It is very hard to differentiate clinically between this seizure and an absence seizure unless an electroencephalogram is recorded at the particular time.

Category III, "unilateral seizures," refers to seizures that affect newborns and young infants and that occur on only one side of the body. These young brains are not yet developed enough for the seizure to become generalized.

Category IV, "unclassified" seizures, refers to those about which there are not enough data to permit otherwise classifying them.

It is important to note that the International Classification deals only with seizure types, not types of epilepsy. Epilepsy is a condition in which a particular patient may have one or several of the various types of seizures. Often the patients with partial-onset seizures will have secondarily generalized tonic-clonic seizures. A patient with petit-mal absence seizures may also occasionally have grand-mal seizures.

Are the seizures painful?

The motor actions and facial expressions of a person having a seizure may appear to an observer as if the seizure is producing pain. However, this is not the case since there are no pain receptors in the brain itself. Some pain fibers are present in the *meninges*, or covering of the brain, and in the larger blood vessels, so that a person may have a headache after a major tonic-clonic seizure.

Are there epilepsies without convulsions? Can a person have more than one type of seizure?

As we've seen, there are many types of seizures that do not have generalized tonic or clonic manifestations. For instance, myoclonic jerks, which may be no more than a single jerk of an arm or a leg, or petit-mal absence seizures are nonconvulsive.

However, recall that a seizure discharge can spread to involve many areas of the brain. Thus a person can have a focal-onset seizure that is only a sensation, a strange feeling, or a jerk, but this may become a partial complex or psychomotor seizure, and, as the discharge spreads to involve the whole brain, may result in a generalized tonic-clonic seizure. Therefore, a person may have several types of seizures, depending on where in the brain the abnormal discharge begins, on how extensive it becomes, and how long it lasts.

I've heard people use the term "aura." What is this?

The *aura* (from the Latin for "air" or "breeze") is the name given to a sensation or feeling that warns of an impending focal-onset seizure. The feeling may be physical or sensory — a tingling, a strange smell; emotional — a feeling of ecstasy; or it may be a heightened sense of one's surroundings; or it may be the experience of déjà vu. The vividness of the aura, especially one of ecstasy or déjà vu, is probably what gave rise to the ancient view of epilepsy as being of supernatural or divine origin.

Physicians today regard the aura as a seizure in and of itself because it is connected with the start of the seizure discharge in a particular area of the brain. In any case, it is caused by the abnormal electrical discharge in the brain, which may then spread to cause complex partial or generalized seizures.

What are lightning seizures?

This is another name for infantile myoclonic and atonic seizures. They are called "lightning" because of their rapid appearance and short duration. Infants affected have been known to have as many as 300 of these seizures a day. One of the major problems connected with rapid seizures is that the infant may fall and sustain an injury.

Some characteristics are often found in babies who have these seizures, although not all of them need be present:

1. Age of six to eighteen months
2. Delayed motor development
3. Poor eating habits
4. Frequent jerking or twitching of muscles
5. Delayed language development and/or mental retardation.

The seizures are extremely difficult to control or to reduce in number.

What are febrile convulsions? Will my child have epilepsy if he has them? Can they cause intellectual or brain damage?

Febrile convulsions are seizures associated with a high body temperature (for example, a rectal temperature of 38°C/101°F or above). They are caused by any illness that is accompanied by a high fever, such as pneumonia, severe sore throat, inner-ear infection, measles, scarlet fever, roseola. Or they may be reactions to high fevers associated with vaccinations or immunizations. Febrile convulsions occur primarily in babies between nine and twenty months old, rarely in those under six months old or over five years. Approximately 5 percent of all infants experience them.

The illnesses causing the high fevers do *not* include central nervous system disorders or organic brain disease, such as meningitis or encephalitis. Acute or chronic diseases of the central nervous system are ruled out in order to distinguish between a febrile convulsion and a seizure disorder. Febrile convulsions are those that occur *only* during a high fever associated with an acute illness *not* originating in the central nervous system.

Of the infants and children who do experience a febrile convulsion, approximately 65 percent never have another seizure of any kind in their lives. Thirty-two percent may have another febrile convulsion. The younger the child experiencing the first febrile convulsion, the greater the risk of recurrence. Among those who have had febrile convulsions, about 5 to 7 percent will develop epilepsy. The likelihood of epilepsy is greatest in those patients who show abnormalities such as slow development or a very long (more than 15 to 30 minutes) first febrile seizure, especially if this one was lateralized or focal-onset in type. The probability of epilepsy is also great in those who show abnormal electroencephalograms.

Although seizure disorders are not directly inherited, the tendency to have febrile convulsions does increase if a close relative has also had them. The incidence of such seizures then increases to about 9 percent. (For more on heredity and seizures, see page 31.)

Immediate treatment varies somewhat according to the individual child and the physician, but involves reduction of the fever by traditional methods (such as sponging or aspirin) and treatment of the underlying infection. The EEG may show a moderate slowing after a seizure but usually returns to "normal" in 7 to 10 days. The use of the EEG, therefore, is usually delayed some 7 to 10 days after a convulsion to detect any continuing abnormal findings.

Long-term anticonvulsive treatment is required for children who experience an extended convulsion or a series of convulsions. There is a controversy over whether previously normal and healthy children who have had a single, short febrile convulsion need to be placed on anticonvulsant medication to prevent future seizures. Most of the literature in this area suggests that such maintenance treatment is not necessary. *If* there is treatment, the physician most probably will use phenobarbital but may use other drugs according to the special needs of the child. Recurring febrile convulsions will require anticonvulsive therapy.

The effects of febrile convulsions are not fully known, though there is some preliminary research evidence that prolonged or frequent convulsions do have an adverse effect on children. Studies have suggested that: (1) children who had several seizures associated with fever during the first year of life tended to perform less well than did their nonaffected siblings on intelligence tests administered later; (2) children with a significantly greater chance of mental retardation were those who had several febrile convulsions on the first day of an illness. However, the reason these children may have early or more frequent febrile seizures may be that there is underlying brain damage existing before any seizure occurred.

In general, single or short febrile convulsions appear to have no lasting effect on the child.

Can you tell me a little more about absence seizures?

Absence seizure is another name for petit mal. It is characterized by a lapse of consciousness that is usually very brief (between 5 and 15 seconds), with an immediate return to alertness at the end of the episode. The patient is not confused as he or she may be after a generalized tonic-clonic seizure, in which the seizure discharge involves the whole brain and causes massive body movements as well as unconsciousness. Dr. J. Kiffin Penry, a leading expert on absence seizures, has shown that there are many small movements associated with them: blinking of the eyes, grinding of the teeth, or other automatic actions.

The brain-wave pattern in patients with absence seizures is quite specific. It is a bilateral spike-and-wave discharge pattern that occurs at about three cycles per second (CPS). Dr. Penry has shown that if the 3-CPS spike-and-wave discharge lasts longer than 1½ seconds, the time it takes for the patient to respond to a flashing light will be increased. Therefore, the patient has a lapse of consciousness, although it may be very brief.

A patient with absence seizures can also have myoclonic or generalized tonic-clonic seizures or both. Approximately 40 to 50 percent of the patients with absence seizures may at some time in their lives experience a generalized tonic-clonic seizure.

The terms *absence variant, petit-mal variant,* and *atypical petit mal* refer to a condition in which there are approximately 1½- to 2½-CPS spike-and-wave discharge patterns. The condition is associated with myoclonic seizures, mental retardation, and a background slowing of the brain waves, as shown on the EEG. It is also referred to as the *Lennox-Gastaut-West syndrome.*

What is post-traumatic epilepsy?

This term refers to persistent seizures that occur *following* a significant injury *(trauma)* to the head. The more serious the injury, the more likely a person is to develop seizures. If the injury is a penetrating wound to the skull that damages the brain directly, the person's chances of having seizures as a result are about 50 percent. If the injury is "closed-head," that is, one with no penetration of the skull, and if it is not severe enough to cause unconsciousness, seizures are very unlikely to develop. The shorter the period of unconsciousness, the lower the incidence of post-traumatic seizures.

What is autonomic epilepsy?

Autonomic seizures, which affect the autonomic nervous system, cause changes in gastrointestinal, circulatory and vasomotor, respiratory, urinary, and sexual behavior. Phenomena such as hypersalivation, repeated swallowing, lip-smacking, chewing, or an abnormal feeling in the epigastric (just below the chest) region of the abdomen, often rising into the throat, can occur. Or the seizure can be one of repeated severe pain in the epigastric region, lasting usually for a few minutes at a time. Circulatory and vasomotor changes include abrupt variation in cardiac rhythm, pallor, flushing and reddening of the skin, or increased perspiration. Respiratory changes may be increased or decreased breathing. Enuretic epileptic seizures are evidenced by a sudden, involuntary loss of urine. A sexual epileptic seizure causes an erection and, extremely rarely, an orgasm. The usual autonomic seizure manifestations generally appear in association with other types of seizures, such as partial complex ones resulting from the spread of the seizure discharge to other parts of the brain.

Why is myoclonic epilepsy often considered separately from the other epilepsies?

The myoclonic epilepsies, which are more common in children, are usually considered as a separate group because of their resistance to conventional treatment by anticonvulsant drugs and the existence of a genetic form of the disorder. The incidence of myoclonic epilepsy is rather rare, occurring in only about 5 percent of those children known to have epilepsy. Approximately two thirds of the cases of myoclonic seizures occur in children under the age of four. The seizures are identifiable by muscle spasms of the eyelids, neck, and arms.

Myoclonus is believed to occur with a sudden electrical discharge from the motor control centers in the midbrain, brainstem, and spinal cord. The discharge may then spread to higher centers of the brain. Myoclonic seizures can occur alone or in association with akinetic, atonic, petit-mal absence, or generalized tonic-clonic seizures. Severe myoclonic seizures often accompany conditions of diffuse brain encephalopathy. Some degree of mental retardation is common.

What is a hysterical seizure?

A hysterical seizure (or pseudoseizure) refers to a seizurelike episode that is not related to an actual electrical discharge in the brain. The phenomenon does not usually come from a conscious effort to deceive, but rather is an unconscious mechanism on the part of the patient for increased attention. Hysterical seizures frequently occur in young women; psychiatric consultation is in order when the seizures become persistent. Most often these seizures appear in patients who also have real seizures; the two can be difficult to tell apart.

What is "kindling"?

It is known that repeated electrical stimulation of parts of the brain in animals can produce spontaneous seizurelike discharges that resemble those of epilepsy. This process is termed *kindling,* meaning that the one ignites the other. It suggests that seizures may bring on, or kindle, more seizures unless they are checked. Although kindling has been demonstrated experimentally in animals, it is still only theoretical in humans, and more research is required.

What is status epilepticus?

A person is in status epilepticus when a series of seizures occurs with no time in between for recovery. Status epilepticus can occur in many types of seizures, including generalized tonic-clonic, absence, partial complex, unilateral, and focal-motor types. When a person experiences continuous absence seizures, it is called *petit-mal status.* When one has continuous focal-motor seizures, it is called *epilepsia partialis continua.*

The most serious form of status epilepticus is a continuous series of generalized tonic-clonic (prolonged grand-mal) seizures without any time for recovery. The patient requires immediate emergency hospitalization. Treatment involves specific anticonvulsant therapy to stop the seizures as quickly as possible, fluids, and emergency medical care.

Approximately 3 percent of adults with epilepsy and 5 to 8 percent of children will undergo at least one episode of status epilepticus. Status occurs most frequently if the patient does not take his medication, especially if he stops abruptly. From 8 to 41 percent of patients who have status will die from it. Those who survive it are felt to have a greater chance of increased seizure frequency, different types of seizures, and some permanent brain damage.

Do seizures get worse with age?

In general, the frequency of seizures continues at about the same rate as one gets older. At times it improves and at other times it worsens. With anticonvulsant therapy, seizure frequency should diminish. One study of patients with petit-mal absence seizures alone showed that approximately 78 percent were seizure-free in five years. But the same study showed that of those patients who have *both* absence and tonic-clonic seizures, only 36 percent were free of the absence seizures in the five-year period. The type and the combination of seizures, therefore, seem to be important in the prognosis.

Are strokes a form of epilepsy?

No. Strokes are brought on by a change in the blood flow to the brain. A stroke can be caused by a *thrombosis* (clotting) in a cerebral artery or by an *embolus* (a small particle from some other area of the body) entering the cerebral blood vessels or by a hemorrhage in the brain. Strokes can look somewhat like seizures, particularly if they are brief and transient: the decrease in the blood flow to the brain can at times last only a few minutes. Sometimes strokes are related to trauma to the blood vessels leading to the brain, especially those in the neck. They can also be caused by malformations of the arteries and veins, called *arteriovenous malformations (AVMs)*. Although most strokes occur in older people, children can have them, too.

In a stroke, the function of the involved area of the brain *decreases,* leading, for example, to a weakness on one side of the body. In most seizures, the function of the brain area *increases,* leading to an action like the jerking of an arm. However, the outward manifestation of a stroke involving the sensory cortex in the parietal lobe can be similar to that resulting from a seizure discharge in the same brain area.

The AVMs that can cause strokes can also cause seizures because they act as irritative foci. It is possible that both a cerebral hemorrhage — a stroke — and a seizure can happen to the same person because of an AVM. Furthermore, strokes in and of themselves, whether they are hemorrhagic or thrombotic, can cause an irritative focus to develop in a brain area that eventually leads to seizures.

My child has lost consciousness after holding his breath. It appeared that he was having a seizure. Could these "attacks" develop into actual seizures?

Infants often have periods of holding their breath after a long period of crying. The cause of breath-holding is not clear, other than that it often follows a prolonged crying spell arising from pain or frustration. If the infant should hold his breath (usually after exhaling) for a long enough time, he may actually lose consciousness. Frequently urination and muscle-jerking follow, and other symptoms outwardly resembling a tonic-clonic seizure. The "attack" is usually over in ten or fifteen seconds.

The episodes are not as dangerous as they appear, and no action on the part of the parents is needed. Unless there are secondary gains or rewards to the child, such as a disproportionate amount of attention or anxiety on the parents' part, the attacks are usually normally outgrown long before the child reaches school age. There is no relationship to epilepsy, or any other undesirable side effects, other than the child's recognition that the episodes may become attention-getters.

Can fainting spells or other conditions be confused with epilepsy in a child?

It is not infrequent that a child without epilepsy may manifest some of the behavioral symptoms often associated with epilepsy. Recurrent episodes of fainting are often initially considered as possible epilepsy. The same is true for breath-holding spells and temper tantrums, which are also often seen in young children and infants. In an emotional upset, a child may cry and then hold the breath until the lips turn blue (cyanosis), which may be followed by fainting. A condition resembling a convulsion may or may not appear. Epilepsy, however, occurs spontaneously without crying, and the cyanosis appears only *after* a convulsion.

An evaluation must be completed to differentiate the conditions. In this case, an EEG is useful in the diagnosis, since the EEG is normal in fainting and breath-holding spells, while abnormalities will usually be revealed in seizure conditions. There is, of course, no need for anticonvulsant medication in fainting or breath-holding conditions.

Older children or adults may have bodily symptoms such as headaches, vomiting spells, or abdominal pains, which are also occasionally confused with epilepsy. These symptoms need an intensive evaluation to rule out the possibility that they may be behavioral manifestations of epilepsy.

If my child has epilepsy, is his overall development likely to be delayed?

Development is a broad concept that refers to every area of the child's growth pattern, such as motor, speech, cognition, and the like. The child with epilepsy does not necessarily develop at a slower rate than other children; however, certain areas of development sometimes tend to be delayed. It is noted in clinical practice that many anticonvulsant medications produce a general blunting of affect, but research on the effects of anticonvulsants on development has not been extensive. One drug, phenobarbital, has been shown to slow cognitive development and physical reaction time in some children.

Through the years, authorities in child development, such as Gesell, Piaget, Cattell, and Bayley, have agreed as to the various ages at which a child normally arrives at certain developmental "milestones." These ages, however, fail to account for the vast individual differences. Because of these differences, it is unfair to compare one child with another on developmental scales. The *sequence* of the developmental skills acquired, however, is far more apt to be correct than the various ages. If your child has epilepsy, he may or may not have reached these milestones at the most common age. To give the parent an approximate idea of the rate of development of the child, the following partial list of motor development is included (taken from A. Attwell, 1973):

		Approximate Age in Weeks
1.	Lifts head when held to adult's shoulder	3
2.	Adjusts position when lifted	4
3.	Holds head erect (unsteadily) when held in upright position	4
4.	Holds head erect and steady when in upright position	8
5.	Lifts upper torso by arms, in prone position	14
6.	Sits with support	15
7.	Lifts head and shoulders when lying on back	19
8.	Sits with slight support	20
9.	Sits alone momentarily with rounded shoulders	22
10.	Sits erect briefly	29
11.	Stands alone by holding furniture	31
12.	Rests on thighs, lower abdomen, and hands	36
13.	Moves from prone position to sitting	44
14.	Pulls self to knees	44
15.	Pulls self to standing position	47
16.	Creeps	47
17.	Walks with help from adult	48
18.	Stands alone without support	54
19.	Walks alone unsupported	60
20.	Walks sideways	66
21.	Climbs stairs or chair	72
22.	Walks backward	76
23.	Goes up and down stairs	120
24.	Stands momentarily on one foot	120

The development of speech and language is a far more cultural-intellectual process than a purely developmental skill such as walking, and is perhaps most affected by epilepsy. Speech is controlled by several "speech centers" in the brain and in this sense is physiological. However, once the functioning of these centers is established, the development of speech patterns becomes an intellectual matter. Remember that no two children are exactly alike; thus the acquisition of speech in terms of norms or averages is difficult to predict. Unlike walking, which can be learned at any time (even

when children have had their legs bound for the first two years of
life, as seen in the Dennis Hopi Indian Studies), there seems to be a
general age at which children *must* learn to talk if they are to speak
normally. The child who has not learned to communicate verbally
by the age of three and a half to four often does not learn to speak
normally *at all*. The child usually follows a specific sequence in the
development of language. Although the major investigators into the
development of speech (Gesell, Thompson, Chen and Irwin, etc.) do
not agree on the specific age at which the various stages occur, they
do agree on the following sequence of verbal skills:

	Approximate Age in Weeks
1. Cries with meaningless frontal vowels ("a," "e," "i")	4
2. Cries in relation to definite body needs	8–12
3. Chuckles audibly	12
4. Coos	12
5. Laughs	15
6. Vocalizes "da"	36
7. Vocalizes "ma"	44
8. Repeats first syllable ("ma-ma," "da-da," etc.)	46
9. Makes "b" sound	48
10. Says first word	50
11. Says two words	52
12. Says three or more connected words	53

It is interesting to note that though the initial attempts at
verbalizing are in small and gradual steps, once the concept of a
meaningful vocabulary has been established (at about one year), the
growth in vocabulary is amazingly rapid.

	Approximate Number of Words
1. One year	3
2. One year, three months	19
3. One year, six months	22

4. One year, nine months	120
5. Two years	275
6. Two years, six months	450
7. Three years	900
8. Three years, six months	1,225
9. Four years	1,550
10. Four years, six months	1,970
11. Five years	2,070
12. Five years, six months	2,290
13. Six years	2,550

To repeat our original statement, the child with epilepsy may or may not be delayed in any of these areas. If he *is,* the likelihood is that the delay is most noticeable in areas involving motor and speech skills. The delay need not necessarily be considered permanent, for children with the proper medical control tend to approximate the norm more closely as they grow older.

Do seizure disorders cause poor coordination?

No. Seizures are symptoms of a dysfunction in the brain, but seizures themselves do not produce subsequent difficulty in muscle control. Poor motor coordination may be the result of a general delay in the child's motor development. It may also be one part of a combination of problems associated with a specific learning disability, which may include hyperactivity, perceptual difficulties, clumsiness, poor balance, and poor fine-motor movements, such as handwriting.

However, during periods of medication adjustment, certain side effects may cause coordination and balance problems. (See Chapter 5, Anticonvulsants.)

Is there a relationship between epilepsy and criminal acts?

Essentially, no. Early writers, under the influence of the description of "criminal types" that Cesare Lombroso published in 1889, assumed that the person with epilepsy was more prone to violence, antisocial behavior, and crime than a normal person. Their writings were largely based on individual cases rather than on group statistics. Modern, carefully controlled studies show that the incidence of criminal acts committed by people who have seizures is no higher than that in the general population, and the old idea that persons with epilepsy commit crimes during seizures is a myth.

Bagley (1971) found a slight incidence of "early environmental and other possible social factors influencing delinquency in epileptics and controls"; he feels that early social as well as neurological factors might account for the development of delinquency among young people with epilepsy. He summarizes that the evidence is weak and of little consequence. Bagley also found that "there is no suggestion of violent or sexual crimes being overrepresented in epileptics in prison." But there is a slightly higher incidence of epilepsy among prisoners; Bagley feels that social factors such as prejudice and employment difficulties may account for this. It is possible that a prisoner is more likely to have had a head injury at some time and that this may also play a role.

King and Young (1978) found the incidence of seizure disorders among prisoners in Illinois to be three times greater than among "middle-class non-prisoner populations." They argue for improved special programs and resources for the detection, treatment, and follow-up of seizure disorders among prisoners.

Is epilepsy related in any way to sexuality?

There is a slight relationship between sexuality and temporal lobe epilepsy, though the relationship is considered more psychological than physiological. A slightly lower sex drive and sporadic impotence and frigidity have been found among those affected by seizure disorders. These conditions are believed to be related not so much to the physical components of epilepsy as to the fears of a seizure during the sex act. Seizures have sometimes been triggered by anxiety during or directly preceding the act. Other than this, epilepsy does not affect one's sexual interest or performance.

Is the suicide rate higher among persons with epilepsy than in the general population?

Various studies have shown that the suicide rate among persons with epilepsy is far higher than that among persons who do not have the disorder. The consensus is that the person with epilepsy frequently suffers from anxiety and depression, and that the rate of suicide (or suicidal attempts) is nearly double that of the normal population.

Gunn (1969) studied suicide attempts of prisoners with epilepsy, and found that 39 percent of the prisoners with epilepsy had made one or more attempts at suicide, as opposed to 22 percent of nonepileptic prisoners. He found the highest rates among those with (1) temporal lobe and (2) "untreatable" epilepsy.

Are persons with epilepsy susceptible to psychological or psychiatric illnesses?

The incidence of psychiatric problems in persons with epilepsy appears to be higher than that of the general population, as might be expected. This does not necessarily mean a direct relationship between epilepsy and neuroses or psychoses. Many psychiatrists believe that certain psychoses, mainly those considered to be manic-depressive and/or schizophrenic, have their origin in physiochemical disturbances in the brain and suggest that a particular chemical disturbance can cause both epilepsy and psychosis in certain susceptible individuals.

Difficulty in coping with the condition and the array of social and family problems can also lead to development of major psychological disorders in some individuals. Furthermore, for some patients irritability and depression occur when seizures are suppressed, or precede a seizure by several days and disappear with its advent.

A special type of psychosis in persons with temporal lobe epilepsy has been described. This involves acute psychotic episodes with prominent schizophrenic-like features, which can last for several days or weeks. It is probable that the patient with psychomotor epilepsy is at higher risk for associated psychiatric disorders than persons with other forms of epilepsy.

Are personality disorders necessarily associated with epilepsy?

There is no evidence of specific personality characteristics among all persons with epilepsy; the same range and degree of personality traits can be found among persons with epilepsy as among the general population. There are, however, some situations created by having epilepsy that can bring about emotional disturbances. Reactions to the seizure condition — such as worry over the threat of an impending seizure; a view of oneself as "different"; depression and feelings of guilt — may cause various forms of atypical behavior. Should these persist, personality disorders may develop. They are, nevertheless, purely individual reactions to one's psychosocial environment.

There has been much recent research on personality and the brain, with interesting findings. Ornstein (1975), citing Sperry, and others have established the fact that each hemisphere of the brain appears to have its own sensations, thoughts, memories, and acts independently of the other. The left hemisphere operates rationally with logical thought and language. The right hemisphere works intuitively and appears to be the center for creativity and nonverbal communication. Thus, an injury to a particular part of the brain can result in certain behavioral characteristics.

Most of the research into personality and the brain has concentrated on temporal lobe epilepsy. Though the evidence thus far has been conflicting, some researchers have found a greater incidence of psychosis with temporal lobe epilepsy than in other forms. Bear and Fedio (1976) recently found differences in emotional expression for those with temporal lobe spikes in the two hemispheres. Persons with left temporal lobe epilepsy tended to focus an ideational pattern of behavioral traits (for example, religious or philosophical interests). Those with the right temporal lobe affected displayed overly emotional behavior.

There is some evidence that persons with epilepsy often show a relatively higher incidence of social aggressiveness. This is found more frequently among males than females. It has also been found that the earlier the onset of epilepsy, the more likely it is that the aggressiveness will develop later. Most authorities believe that if aggression does exist in persons with epilepsy more than in the general population, it is associated more with social disadvantage and learning problems than with epilepsy itself.

Do people with epilepsy tend to behave in similar ways? In short, is there a "personality type" for epilepsy?

No, as was mentioned, though this was not always considered so. There have been prejudices and misconceptions for years concerning people with virtually every condition, such as the "personality type" of the intellectually gifted, the "Down's Syndrome type," and so on. Only a generation ago, the psychoanalytic view of the "epileptic personality" was widely held. As recently as 1950, two English researchers reported that people with epilepsy tended to have what they termed an "existing epileptic makeup," and as a group were considered to have either specific or "miscellaneous personality disorders" solely because they had epilepsy.

It is the authors' opinion that no such thing as the "epileptic personality type" exists, any more than that there is an epileptic mentality. People with epilepsy, like everyone else, react to their own problems in varying ways. Despite a number of studies in this area, no clear evidence exists to suggest a type of personality or set of behavior traits that is unique to persons with epilepsy as a group.

2

WHAT CAUSES EPILEPSY?

What causes epilepsy?

Epilepsy is a symptom, not a disease in and of itself. A seizure is a physical manifestation of something wrong in the brain cortex that causes an excessive electrical discharge in the neurons of the brain. Consequently, anything that affects the cortex of the brain, which contains the bulk of the neurons, can cause changes that eventually may result in a seizure disorder. Some etiologic factors are:

1. Brain damage before or at birth (for example, congenital malformation, anoxia, fetal infection)
2. Head trauma significant enough to injure the brain and cause a scar formation
3. Infections, such as meningitis or encephalitis, that have left some scarring of the brain
4. Metabolic disorders that also affect brain functions (for example, phenylketonuria)
5. Brain tumors
6. Parasitic infections that can leave cysts on the brain
7. Strokes, which can be brought on by either decreased blood supply to the brain or hemorrhage into or around the brain

8. Degenerative brain disease
9. Genetic disorders
10. Toxic conditions resulting in brain disorder (for example, kernicterus, lead poisoning)

Hypoglycemia (low blood sugar), hypocalcemia (low blood calcium), and hypomagnesia (low blood magnesium) separately or together can cause seizures in newborns, but are very rarely associated with seizures in adults. Pyridoxine (vitamin B_6) deficiency may also cause seizures in infants. In adults, there may be contributing factors that lead to seizures. For example, chronic alcoholics may tend to fall and thus risk head trauma. Sudden withdrawal from alcohol by an alcoholic may precipitate seizures. Abuse of other drugs, such as barbiturates, cocaine, and Quaaludes, may bring about seizures, particularly when the drugs are suddenly withdrawn.

In about 70 to 80 percent of the cases of epilepsy a definitive cause is not found. These cases are called *idiopathic*, which means arising from no known cause. Presumptive causes, however, can be determined by looking at the *age* of the onset of seizures. If an infant from birth to two years old develops seizures, the presumptive cause is birth injury or degenerative brain disease. If a child or young adult from ages two to twenty develops seizures, the cause most likely is related to congenital birth injury, febrile thrombosis in an artery leading to the brain, head trauma, or an infection, such as meningitis or encephalitis. In adults aged twenty to thirty-five, the most frequent cause is head trauma, but *neoplasm* (tumor) should also be considered. During middle age (thirty-five to fifty-five), brain tumor, head trauma, and strokes lead the list. In the older age group (fifty-five and over), strokes and tumors are the most likely causes. Screening with the computerized brain scanner (see page 65), for example, has revealed that about 10 percent of those with epilepsy had previously undiagnosed brain tumors. Brain tumor should be considered a presumptive cause when an adult who has never had seizures before suddenly develops focal-onset seizures.

Certainly it becomes apparent in studying seizure disorders that one of the most frequent causes (particularly of those disorders that persist throughout life) is brain damage, occurring in the womb or during birth. Injury during the birth process may cause bleeding inside or on the surface of the brain, or may bruise the brain tissue, causing swelling or even destroying the tissue. Lack of oxygen during birth may result in loss of nerve cells. These conditions may not be immediately apparent but may result in the onset of seizures months later. To prevent seizures, therefore, thorough prenatal and postnatal care of the infant and the mother is of the utmost importance.

Given the fact that so many epilepsies are idiopathic, there is a desperate need for further research about the causes of this "most neglected" of all disorders.

What causes the seizure itself?

As we have seen, the human brain has a normal, ongoing, controlled electrical activity, at certain set frequencies and with interaction of neurons in various brain centers. When this activity gets out of control and an excessive electrical discharge takes place in the brain, a seizure occurs. Anyone can have a seizure under specific stressful circumstances, but exactly what triggers a seizure in a particular individual at a particular time is not absolutely understood. It seems to have something to do with the susceptibility of that person to stress and a tendency toward abnormal electrical discharge in the brain. The type of seizure, as we have discussed, is determined by the area of the brain involved in the seizure discharge, the extent of the discharge, and its duration.

Is epilepsy inherited?

The role of heredity in seizure disorders is still not completely understood and has been debated by authorities for many years. Epilepsy seems to fall along a spectrum, with totally acquired epilepsy at one end and almost purely genetic forms at the other. Most epilepsies seem to be in the middle of the spectrum. There is considerable evidence that genetic factors are involved in a predisposition toward epilepsy and in specific types of brain waves among those who have it.

In assessing the hereditary factors, one should first consider the risk of having seizures to the population in general. One study shows the overall risk that a newborn will develop recurrent seizures by age ten is 0.7 percent; 1 percent by age twenty; and 1.7 percent by age forty. The risk becomes higher for the siblings (brothers and sisters) of patients who have seizures. Studies show that if the patient developed the seizures before the age of four, the risk was approximately 7.5 percent that the siblings would develop seizures by the age of twenty. If the patient's seizures began between the ages of four and fifteen, the risk that siblings would develop seizures was 4.3 percent by the age of twenty and 8 percent by the age of forty. In other words, the older the patient was when his seizures began, the less likely it is that the siblings will also have seizures.

Another study, of patients who had generalized-onset seizures, particularly petit-mal absence seizures, shows that the risk of a sibling's also having seizures was approximately 8 percent. If one of the patient's parents also had absence seizures, the risk to the siblings was then 13 percent. Of particular interest in these studies is the fact that 37 percent of the siblings of patients with seizures had EEG abnormalities — a percentage much higher than that for the general population. Only about 25 percent of the siblings with the abnormal EEGs also actually had seizures, however.

This same question, is epilepsy inherited, is asked by patients with seizures in regard to *their* children. The data are difficult to obtain, obviously, because studies must be long-term, with careful follow-up. Those that have been made seem to indicate that if a parent has an idiopathic, generalized-onset seizure disorder, such as petit-mal absence seizures, the risk to his or her child is between 4.4 and 11 percent. If the seizures are the acquired type, particularly focal-onset, the risk is between 1.6 and 3.2 percent.

Another aspect of the heredity question has to do with epilepsy in one or both parents. When one parent has petit-mal absence seizures, the overall risk is about 8 percent. The probability that the child will have seizures is a little higher if the parent with epilepsy is the mother rather than the father. If both parents have epilepsy, however, the risk to their children rises sharply, to an estimated 25 to 30 percent. Some authorities estimate it as high as 50 percent. This risk is greater if parents have a generalized-onset seizure disorder rather than a focal-onset type, such as psychomotor epilepsy.

It is important for couples with epilepsy to utilize genetic counseling, in order to gain specific information about their own situation and the understanding needed to make an informed choice regarding children. If there is a family history of epilepsy or if a previous child has epilepsy or any other central nervous system disorder, or if one or both parents have epilepsy that began in infancy, then a genetic work-up and estimation of specific risk factors are advised. Genetic counseling may be arranged through the family physician or by contacting the local medical society or nearest medical school.

Can seizures in a newborn infant be caused by drug addiction of the mother?

Unfortunately, this is true — drugs are a frequent cause of infantile seizures. Many pregnant women who have taken heroin, morphine, or excessive alcohol or have sniffed glue have produced infants with a "narcotic withdrawal symptom." The condition in an infant is often serious and has been known to be fatal if not treated early.

Is it dangerous for a pregnant woman to smoke?

No direct relationship between smoking during pregnancy and epilepsy in the offspring has been found. However, there is a positive relationship between smoking during pregnancy and the weight of the baby at birth. The average birth weight of these babies is 8 ounces less than that of babies born to non-smoking mothers.

Clinical evidence shows that smoking predisposes a pregnant woman to premature labor, which is often a cause of low birth weight, and premature babies who are prone to respiratory illness with resulting anoxia (lack of oxygen) and subsequent seizures. Smoking during pregnancy should be avoided, especially by a woman who has had a previous miscarriage.

Can a parent's beating a child cause epilepsy?

The problem of the battered child is far more common than is generally recognized. A nervous mother or father may love the infant and have no intention of causing permanent brain damage, but may strike the infant or child on the face or head in sudden anger, resulting in trauma to the brain. Any blow that is of sufficient strength to produce unconsciousness or a skull fracture can cause hemorrhage of the blood vessels on the surface of or inside the brain, leading to brain injury, abnormal electrical discharges, and possible seizures. This "battered child syndrome" accounts for an estimated 2,500 deaths per year in the United States alone, and for six times that number with skull malformations, mental retardation, or epilepsy.

Is epilepsy contagious?

At one time in our history it was believed that seizure disorders could be transmitted from one person to another by way of the saliva, which is often freely discharged through drooling during a seizure. Another common belief was that the disorder was respiratory in origin and was therefore contagious when one was in close contact with the affected person. None of these beliefs is true, and epilepsy is in no way contagious.

Is birth order a factor in epilepsy?

The firstborn are more likely to have epilepsy than subsequent children. This has been documented repeatedly by research studies, though the reason is not clear. It has been suggested that the prevalence of epilepsy among the firstborn may be explained at least partly by physiological factors, such as the pelvic size of the new mother, inasmuch as the firstborn also tend to have a higher incidence of birth injuries.

Birth order seems to have the greatest significance in temporal lobe epilepsy. One study found that 60 percent of those with temporal lobe epilepsy were firstborn.

If head injuries cause epilepsy so frequently, can it be prevented in those cases?

It is true that head injury is a frequent cause. As we have seen, if the injury actually penetrates the brain, the risk of having seizures is about 50 percent. In about 25 percent of the cases, however, seizures after the injury do not become recurrent. Also, approximately 50 percent of post-traumatic seizures stop after about eight years. In closed-head injuries, the risk of post-traumatic seizures is much less, about 5 percent. The variations in these frequencies depend upon the penetration of the brain and the length of any period of unconsciousness. If the patient is unconscious for less than 24 hours, does not have any seizures within the first month, and shows no signs of focal neurological damage, there is then less than a 5 percent chance of developing post-traumatic epilepsy.

Some evidence exists that post-traumatic epilepsy can be prevented by use of the drug dexamethasone, which decreases brain swelling after an injury. The overall survival rate following head injury has improved with the use of this drug. Some physicians also start anticonvulsant medications immediately after a head injury, but just how effective they are in preventing post-traumatic seizures is still a matter of controversy. Recent studies indicate that phenobarbital in the blood at therapeutic levels may be effective, but more research is still being done on this matter.

Since there are an estimated 20,000 *new* cases of epilepsy each year in the United States as a result of head injury, prevention of the injuries clearly means prevention of epilepsy. Automobile accidents lead the list of causes of injury. The Commission for the Control of Epilepsy and Its Consequences estimates that the implementation of its automobile safety recommendations (mandatory helmets for motorcyclists, 55-mile-per-hour speed-limit enforcement, mandatory seat and shoulder straps, etc.) in the United States could save more than $600,000,000 in costs of epilepsy alone, not to mention the cost in lives and in suffering by those who have epilepsy as a result of head injuries.

There have been many instances of adults having post-traumatic seizures who have never experienced any seizures before. The psychological aspects of this situation seem to be more difficult to control than the seizures themselves. The adult frequently has more difficulty accepting the fact that he has a seizure disorder than the person who has grown up with the condition. Even more complex are the paroxysmal disorders without convulsions that may follow a trauma to the brain, and that frequently cause the person to think of himself as emotionally disturbed or even psychotic.

Can infections cause epilepsy?

More than 25 percent of those with acquired (organic) epilepsy have developed it as a result of an infection. The infection can be either a meningitis (an inflammation of the meninges that also affects the brain surface), or an encephalitis (an infection involving the brain itself). Though epilepsy may sometimes develop from infections following measles, or mumps, or diphtheria, and the like, it is more common in connection with bacterial meningitis, for which no vaccine has yet been found.

What causes the so-called reflex epilepsies?

Certain seizures, which are most often tonic-clonic or focal in nature, are occasionally triggered by a known and easily identified stimulus. These stimuli are sensory in nature, and the victim usually soon becomes aware of his particular sensitivity to one or more of the following:

1. *Seizures induced by flashing lights.* This condition, known as photosensitive or photogenic epilepsy, though rare, is one of the most common of the reflex epilepsies; seizures are easily invoked in those who are sensitive to sudden changes in light patterns. The advent of television, especially when it flickers, has increased the incidence of such seizures in both children and adults. The flickering of sunlight seen through a row of trees as one drives past has historically been another common cause. The writers have known of many children who have induced seizures (deliberately or accidentally) by rapidly moving their fingers before their eyes while looking at a bright light.

2. *Seizures induced by a sudden touch.* This stimulated reflex is

more rare, and it has been debated as to whether it is actually epilepsy. A sudden heavy tap has been known to bring on a focal motor attack in certain people, which in turn causes sudden jerking motions in parts or all of the body. Those who are especially sensitive to this "tactile epilepsy" are often subject to other forms of reflex seizures, and if such is the case, it becomes more likely that the person *does* have epilepsy.

3. *Seizures induced by sudden noises.* Peculiarly, the persons affected by auditory stimuli are usually most sensitive to a particular sound (for instance, music, an explosion), and often tend not to be as sensitive to other sounds of equal intensity. Some authorities consider it possible that the person has an emotional involvement with the particular type of sound. In one such case, the *type* of music (symphonic) triggered the seizure, lending an emotional and associative aspect to these seizures.

4. *Seizures induced by reading.* Certain seizure-prone persons have been known to have seizures more often when they performed tasks that involved the use of their eyes or hands while engaged in the thinking process (for example, reading rapidly, playing chess, working an arithmetic problem). It is not definitely known whether the primary stimulus is the eye-hand coordination, such as pointing with the finger while reading, or writing by longhand or typewriter, or whether it is the combination of thinking in connection with rapid eye movements. Some have recognized their particular sensitivity to this type of stimulus and have learned to avoid reading rapidly or using a combination of kinesthetic tasks.

Can people deliberately bring seizures on themselves? If so, why?

Self-induced seizures are not uncommon. Some people do it deliberately; others are apparently unaware of any involvement in contributing to a seizure. Persons have been known to trigger seizures by their own will without any known physical stimulus. Similarly, some rare individuals have been able to control their seizures by the same method, and this group has been of special interest to physicians as a means of helping other people avoid the onset of a seizure.

Others, usually children, have been able to cause a seizure by using a particular reflex stimulus (for example, a flashing light) that they know precipitates an attack. Some people can bring about seizures by hyperventilation under stress. Children may use seizures as an escape mechanism or a means to gain attention; so, occasionally, may some adults. They may find that there are advantages to having seizures, such as getting increased attention from persons important to them, being cared for, or avoiding responsibilities expected of them that they do not feel capable of handling. For these individuals, the benefits of seizures outweigh all the negative consequences.

Failure to take medication regularly is also seen in some patients who wish to have some seizures so that they may continue to be regarded as handicapped and thereby also continue to receive medical or disability benefits.

Are there conditions that increase the frequency of seizures?

In patients with a tendency to have seizures, there are often certain precipitating factors. Sleep deprivation, for example, is one. Attendants in the emergency rooms of college infirmaries can often tell when final exams are being given because one or two students may come in after experiencing their first generalized tonic-clonic seizures — provoked by getting only one or two hours of sleep for several nights in a row. It is generally felt that the seizure patient should get about seven or eight hours of sleep each night in order to avoid this problem.

Alcohol withdrawal can frequently precipitate seizures in patients who are already susceptible to them. In general, if one drinks enough to become drunk, one is much more likely to have a seizure some twelve to twenty-four hours later. This is also true for sudden withdrawal from several other drugs.

Women often have more seizures just before or in the early days of the menstrual period. Emotional stress, fatigue, or major illnesses, particularly those associated with high fever, are also likely to increase seizure frequency. Absence seizures can be brought on by hyperventilation. Indeed, a physician may ask a patient to hyperventilate deliberately in order to bring on such a seizure and thus verify that the patient has typical petit-mal absence seizures.

When there has been so much profitable research on other disorders, why has there been so little on epilepsy?

Actually, there *has* been a great deal of research on the basic mechanisms of epilepsy and on the treatment of seizure disorders. In the past, however, financial support for epilepsy research has been relatively low, primarily because no great public pressure for funding the research has been put on Congress. There have always been very active lobbies for relatively rare diseases, such as muscular dystrophy, because sufferers from those diseases and their relatives have been active and outspoken. Too often, in the case of epilepsy, parents and patients have felt that the disorder is a "bad mark" on the family and have therefore tried to keep it hidden. If significant progress is to be made in epilepsy research there will have to be organized, vocal pressure like that for the other, more "popular" diseases. It is important for those with seizure disorders and their families to let their elected officials know how they feel about increasing the effectiveness of treating the condition. Research funding is usually directly proportionate to the degree of public pressure. As more and more who suffer from or are affected by epilepsy come forward to let their congressmen know about the needs, greater support for research will be given and more rapid progress made in the knowledge about and treatment of seizure disorders.

3

HOW PREVALENT IS EPILEPSY?

How many people have epilepsy?

It is difficult to determine the exact number of people who have epilepsy. Seizures can be concealed, and except during an attack a person may show no indication of the disorder. Many people have epilepsy that is not diagnosed, and some persons do not seek or continue medical treatment. Furthermore, there are variations in the numbers known to health agencies in different parts of the country. As a result, the prevalence of epilepsy is most probably greatly underestimated.

Studies of the prevalence of epilepsy in the United States and other countries yield estimates that depend on many factors, such as the definition of epilepsy chosen by the investigator, the degree of severity, and whether only the cases recognized by health agencies are included. Not all cases of epilepsy are active at all times. Estimates of the prevalence rate in the United States range from 6.57 cases per 1,000 to 18.6 cases per 1,000. The major study (Hauser and Kurland, 1975) utilized a comprehensive survey of medical and hospital records in Rochester, Minnesota, indicating a rate of 6.57 *identified active* cases of epilepsy per 1,000 persons. The study covered all ages and used tight criteria for seizure disorders. A study by Rose (1973) in Maryland yielded a prevalence rate of 18.6 per 1,000, though this included cases with complex febrile convulsions. Investigators from other countries show rates of 6.2 per 1,000 in England, 4.1 per 1,000 in Israel, and 3.5 per 1,000 in Norway.

While the rate of known seizure disorders is difficult to assess, the rate of those unknown is even more elusive. At present, there is no accurate method of determining the degree of underestimation of the prevalence rates. Two studies, conducted by Meighan in Oregon and by Rose in Maryland, provide some information about the number of cases that might be unknown to the health care systems. Both investigators surveyed the seizure disorders evidenced among third graders and conducted neurological examinations of a sample of these children. Of children who had convulsive disorders, Meighan found that 24.1 percent and Rose found that 19.8 percent had not had any medical contact! From these data, it may be estimated that perhaps 20 percent of all children with epilepsy have not been medically identified.

From the prevalence rate and underestimate rate, it is possible to estimate the number of cases of epilepsy in the United States. These estimates vary from a figure of 2,135,000 to 4,000,000 persons, or between 1 and 2 percent of the population. The Commission for the Control of Epilepsy and Its Consequences concluded that there were approximately 2,135,000 Americans with *active epilepsy* — those with seizures not under control in the past five years or those being treated with anticonvulsants.

The commission was conservative in its figures and reports this number as an *under*estimate of the total number of persons with epilepsy in the United States. When the known active, the unreported, and the unknown cases are combined, the total number of persons with epilepsy in the country is probably between 3,000,000 and 4,000,000.

Epilepsy represents one of the most common neurological disorders in the United States and presumably in the world. The estimated numbers of cases of neurological disorders in the United States, based upon data from the National Institute of Neurological and Communicative Disorders and Stroke, are as follows:

Mental retardation (not always neurological)	6,000,000
Epilepsy	2,135,000–4,000,000
Parkinson's disease	1,000,000

Cerebral palsy	750,000
Multiple sclerosis (and related diseases)	500,000
Muscular dystrophy	250,000
Huntington's disease	50,000
Myasthenia gravis	30,000

If we include all the other related neurological dysfunctions, there would be an estimated 20,000,000 cases in the United States alone. Neurological disorders account for one out of every five cases of hospitalization, and for one of every five deaths in the United States. As can be seen from the above list, epilepsy probably affects more persons than Parkinson's disease, cerebral palsy, multiple sclerosis, and muscular dystrophy combined!

As mentioned, there are undoubtedly vast numbers of persons whose seizures are controlled to the extent that they are able to conceal their condition from the general public. Many people with epilepsy are reluctant to admit their disorder for fear of social or economic repercussions. They realize that the general public may give lip service to acceptance of the disorder but inwardly reject it. As a result, if people with epilepsy are *able* to conceal the condition, they often simply *do*. Other disorders such as mental retardation, cerebral palsy, and the like are readily apparent and usually undeniable, but not controlled epilepsy.

Of equal importance is the fact that many retarded individuals, institutionalized or at home, have epilepsy in addition to retardation. Between 200,000 and 300,000 such individuals are so handicapped that they need supervised living arrangements. However, since retardation is the primary diagnosis, these persons are considered as mentally retarded rather than epileptic; thus, the estimated figure could be even higher.

Whatever figure we accept, epilepsy is most certainly a significant disorder in terms of numbers, and has already been established as the most expensive as well as the second most prevalent neurological disorder.

Why am I hearing more about epilepsy than I was a few years ago?

Due to increased dissemination of information, public awareness and understanding of many dysfunctions have increased greatly. Consequently, parents and those individuals who are afflicted are less reluctant to discuss their problems with others.

Consider mental retardation. The incidence of retardation is no greater than it ever was, but when noted personalities or families, such as Pearl Buck, Dale Evans and Roy Rogers, and the Kennedys, to name a few, could publicly write about their retarded children, it no longer seemed necessary for others to attempt to conceal it.

Of even greater importance is the fact that the ancient stigmata of "demon possession" or mental illness once associated with epilepsy have long been debunked. When people with epilepsy can write some of the world's most beautiful music, rank among its greatest scientists, become popular actors, and win statewide beauty contests, others surely no longer need to feel unproductive because of this disorder. Many who once might have hidden the fact that they had epilepsy now feel more comfortable discussing it.

Are seizure disorders more common in young children than in adults?

The incidence of seizure disorders does vary according to age. The greatest number of new cases in relation to the population occurs in the first year of life. The incidence then drops steadily until age sixty, when there is a marked increase. About 75 percent of the cases of epilepsy begin before adulthood. Although epilepsy is less likely to have its onset in adults, it is possible for persons of any age to acquire the disorder.

What is the overall incidence of seizures in young children?

Various studies have reported seizures in young children (before age five) at the surprisingly high incidence of 5 to 7 percent, though the seizure activity of itself is not necessarily epilepsy. Infant seizure disorders represent by far the most common forms of neurological abnormalities. Accurate data on the incidence in infancy and early childhood are sparse and complicated by the questions of definition of epilepsy at that age, and especially by febrile convulsions. As mentioned earlier, the presence of seizures in infants does not necessarily indicate continuing epilepsy.

What percentage of children with seizure disorders may expect to be completely rid of the problem in adulthood?

An estimated 60 percent of all children with seizure disorders who receive proper medical control of the seizures early in life have been found to become seizure-free and require no medication in adulthood. Another 20 percent can attain partial control. The best results have been found when the child had generalized onset tonic-clonic or absence forms.

The recent research study on this subject by Holowach (1972) shows that 76 percent of children were seizure-free when checked eight years after termination of anticonvulsant therapy.

Will my child outgrow his condition?

Many children with mild neurological disorders or minimal brain dysfunction appear to outgrow the condition in their late teens. It is hypothesized that the organizational ability of the brain continues to mature, and, in the case of actual brain injury, the nearby related nondamaged cells of the brain sometimes pick up a part of the function of the damaged cells.

Concerning epilepsy, some children do outgrow their seizures, while others must take medication the rest of their lives. After several years of good control with medication, the physician will normally progressively decrease the dosage under careful monitoring. Eventually, the medication may be stopped (if the seizures do not resume), and the person will be seizure-free without medication. In this sense, he may be considered to have outgrown the condition, though a more accurate term would be "permanent seizure arrest."

What is the overall prognosis for patients with epilepsy?

A recent very thorough study of the prognosis for epilepsy patients was made by the Mayo Clinic in Rochester, Minnesota (Annegers et al., 1979). Through the clinic's records, all diagnosed cases of epilepsy in the population of Rochester between 1935 and 1974 were identified. Patients were considered to have epilepsy if they had had at least two seizures that did not seem to be provoked by an acute cause. The study excluded those who had had only febrile convulsions and those who had had only one seizure without apparent cause.

Remission of epilepsy was defined as a seizure-free period of five years; thus, remission status could not be attained until five years or more after the initial diagnosis. If a patient had one or more seizures after that period, he was considered to have had a relapse. The study also considered the prospect for "successful discontinuance of anticonvulsant medication" in connection with remission. Since the patients considered were those in a general population rather than those from a specialty clinic, the conclusions the study offers about remission and relapse are particularly interesting.

The net probability of being in remission (five years or more without seizures and continuing so) at ten years after the diagnosis was 61 percent; at twenty years, it was 70 percent. In relation to medication, the study showed that "at 20 years after the initial diagnosis . . . , approximately 30 percent of the patients continued to have seizures, approximately 20 percent continued to take anticonvulsant medication but had been free of seizures for at least 5 years, and approximately 50 percent had been without seizures or medication for at least 5 years."

The prognosis also differs according to the causes and types of seizures. For patients whose seizures had no known cause (idiopathic) the probability of being in remission at twenty years was 74 percent. Patients with major neurological problems had a remission probability of 46 percent at twenty years. The probability for those with generalized tonic-clonic seizures was 85 percent; for those with petit-mal absence seizures, 80 percent; and for those with partial complex seizures, 65 percent.

The study also correlated remission and age at the time of diagnosis: "at 10 years after diagnosis, the probability of being in remission was 75 percent for those whose epilepsy was diagnosed before 10 years of age, 68 percent for those diagnosed between ages 10 and 19 . . . , and 63 percent for those with diagnosis between ages 20 and 59 years."

The probability of a relapse in the first five years after entering remission status was 8 percent; 15 percent by the tenth year after remission; and 24 percent by twenty years. The likelihood of relapse increased according to the age at diagnosis. Moreover, "roughly two-thirds of the patients who experience relapse were not taking anticonvulsant medication, but the relapses rarely occurred soon after discontinuance of such medication."

As the authors say in their summary: "The rates for remission we encountered were generally higher than those previously reported. . . . Prognosis for remission . . . is poor in patients with associated neurologic dysfunction identified from birth. Patients with idiopathic seizures and survivors of postnatally acquired epilepsy have better prospects for eventual remission. The probability of remission is highest in patients with generalized-onset seizures diagnosed before 10 years of age. Prognosis is less favorable for those with partial complex seizures and adult-onset epilepsy." In short, the best prognosis is for those with generalized-onset seizures diagnosed at an early age.

Is the incidence of epilepsy on the decrease as a result of the medical progress in the past few decades?

No, on the contrary, it has slightly *increased*. Granted, epilepsy has come under far better control, and many cases have been prevented that might have resulted in serious seizure disorders thirty years ago. Strangely, it has been the very medical progress that has resulted in the increase of the number of persons with epilepsy, for the following reasons:

1. Many infants with congenital cerebral defects who might have died a generation ago can now be saved. Though the

infants' lives have been spared, they represent a far greater risk of having seizure disorders than the normal population.

2. Premature births at one time constituted a vast number of infant mortality cases. These infants are now more easily saved, resulting in a higher incidence of brain damage and epilepsy.

3. Better diagnostic procedures have revealed more early cases of epilepsy and have identified atypical convulsive disorders that were previously undiagnosed or misdiagnosed.

4. Parents of children with epilepsy, as well as the victims themselves, do not feel the same need to hide the affliction that they did a generation ago. Because of increased community understanding, more cases are being reported.

Are persons with epilepsy more likely to be mentally retarded?

The research on this subject has been sparse; however, we could say that there is *no* real evidence through a scientifically controlled study of matched groups that intellectual functioning is lowered because of epilepsy. There is evidence that there *may* be lower functioning when there is brain damage or when seizures begin at an early age and are not subject to control. The earlier in a child's life there is brain damage, the greater the possibility of eventually impaired intellectual functioning. As stated, however, the fact that one has epilepsy does not presuppose mental retardation. There have been too many brilliant people with epilepsy to make such an unwarranted assumption.

There are several primary causes of mental impairment among those with epilepsy who are also retarded (reported by Dr. William Lennox, 1962):

1. Primary congenital defect, in which the seizure disorders are the secondary factor

2. A brain injury that produces both a congenital defect and the seizures

3. Deterioration because of the frequency and severity of seizures
4. Degree of medication (including both overmedication and undermedication).

In children with mental retardation and epilepsy it is important to recognize that brain damage is the primary cause of both conditions. The seizures themselves have not produced the mental retardation.

Parents are often concerned, however, that the seizures themselves will cause mental retardation if they continue. It is generally believed that the abnormal electrical discharges do not actually cause damage to the brain cells. Kindling experiments in animals, wherein very small electrical shocks are administered repeatedly, do show changes in the animals' tendency to have seizures as well as some cellular damage. The relationship of these discoveries to human epilepsy has not been clearly defined, but they raise the possibility that continued seizures may make patients more likely to have future seizures and may cause some mild brain-cell alterations.

Many neurologists believe that severe or prolonged seizures that produce respiratory slowing and therefore reduce oxygen to the brain will cause additional damage. Cases in which there is a decrease in intellectual functioning are rare and are more the result of factors other than the seizures. Even if damage is known to have occurred to some portion of the brain (as from an accident), seizures are not suspected of increasing that damage. In fact, other nondamaged cells tend to take over some of the functions lost by the damaged cells.

Is the incidence of mental retardation greater when a child has a particular type of seizure?

As was stated in the previous question, epilepsy itself does not presuppose mental retardation. However, a relationship between the *type* of seizure disorder and intelligence has been found on a statistical basis when large groups are studied. This means that a person's *chances* of mental subnormality are greater or less, depending on the type of seizures he has, rather than that he automatically falls into a certain intellectual category because of the type of seizure.

Children with petit-mal absence and some generalized tonic-clonic seizure types and psychomotor forms of epilepsy tend to compare well with the general population on intelligence tests. When the child has myoclonic or akinetic seizures, the chances of mental retardation are greater, and even more so when these seizures developed during the first few years of life. Remember that we are speaking statistically rather than individually, and that a blanket statement should not be made.

What is hyperactivity? Is it associated with a seizure disorder?

Hyperactivity is a condition of excessive physical activity found in varying degrees in a large number of children. The hyperkinetic syndrome involves an excessive amount of physical body movement, distractability, impulsiveness, and short attention span. Parents and teachers often comment that the child is "constantly moving," "restless," or "won't stop to listen." There are wide variations in behavior and degree of hyperactivity. The diagnosis should not be assumed merely because the child is active, but should be made by a team including a physician, psychologist, teacher, and educational specialist.

Some children are hyperactive only before a seizure, and their condition is a part of the seizure disorder. Hyperactivity is only a symptom of an emotional or neurological condition in much the same way that a seizure is a symptom of a neurological dysfunction. If the hyperactivity is a result of a neurological dysfunction, the cause may be the same as that which produced the seizures — head injury, infection, genetic condition, and so on. Some children have both a hyperkinetic syndrome and a seizure disorder.

A child who is truly hyperactive has little control over his behavior and has difficulty following directions. Punishment only increases the problem. Most hyperactive children are of normal intelligence. However, a significant number have learning disabilities and require specialized techniques at school. These children frequently develop emotional problems.

An effective educational program, counseling, and a structured home environment are the primary treatments for hyperactivity. Most children respond well to consistent daily routines, and require advance preparation if the routine is to be changed. Some are helped by a medication such as Dexedrine, Ritalin, or Cylert if the hyperactivity is organically caused. The mechanisms by which stimulant drugs work to produce a change in the hyperactive child are unknown. However, if these drugs are going to be effective, the action is usually noticed within two weeks. Medication alone is seldom the answer, and must be combined with appropriate educational therapy, counseling, and environmental changes. For children with seizure disorders *and* hyperactivity, the treatment for hyperactivity may be added to the anticonvulsant therapy.

Are more boys than girls affected by the hyperkinetic syndrome? Do they outgrow the condition?

The reports vary, but approximately 5 to 10 percent of school-age children may be regarded as hyperkinetic. The syndrome is common among both boys and girls with epilepsy, especially when associated with brain damage sustained in the early years. The ratio of boys to girls affected by hyperactivity is about 4 to 1. The reasons for this are not clear, although a number have been proposed to explain the preponderance of boys affected:

1. There are slightly more boys born than girls, by a ratio of about 104 to 100.
2. The ratio of *firstborn* boys over girls is even higher, suggesting the greater possibility of a birth injury (birth injuries are more commonly reported among the firstborn than in subsequent births).
3. The head size of the male offspring at birth is slightly larger than that of the female, increasing the possibility of a birth injury.
4. The male offspring is slightly more susceptible than the female to genetic defects, because of sex-linked (mother-son) inheritance (such as hemophilia, color blindness, baldness, etc.). Frequently, the hyperactive pattern will be similar to that experienced by the fathers.

5. Boys mature at a relatively slower rate than do girls.
6. The social-cultural pressures on young boys to "succeed" and to appear "masculine" produce more stress on boys.

Most hyperactive children will improve with age, and the condition frequently ends during adolescence. If hyperactivity interferes with learning or relationships with family and friends, the child may develop a psychological problem from the condition that is difficult to change. In short, while the child tends to outgrow the hyperactivity, the previously associated learning or behavioral problems may persist and, without treatment, cause needless suffering.

Is it harmful to a woman with epilepsy to become pregnant?

There is no reason to counsel young women with epilepsy not to become pregnant as long as they are under good medical care and seizure control. There are some unique potential problems to pregnant women with epilepsy, however, the major one being an increased susceptibility to seizures. For some women, seizures become worse in either intensity or frequency, especially during the first three months of pregnancy. This is more likely to happen if the seizures were poorly controlled before the pregnancy. The age of the mother or the age at which seizures first occurred is unrelated to increase in seizures during pregnancy. The increase may be related to a lower serum level of anticonvulsant medication caused by the increased metabolism of the pregnant woman.

Some women taking phenytoin (Dilantin) may have a deficiency of folic acid, and their physicians may want to add folic acid to their diets during the pregnancy to prevent folic-acid deficiency anemia and other problems.

Although precautions must be taken, it is indeed possible for a woman with epilepsy to have children. Any decision regarding pregnancy should be made with the advice of the physician, who will consider the mother's health, the presence of the disorder in other members of the immediate family, the level of the mother's seizure control, and the ability of the parents to care for and rear a child.

Does anticonvulsant medication increase the risk of fetal abnormalities?

The answer to this question is complex. Studies of a large population of women with seizures indicate that the incidence of fetal abnormalities is higher among them than that among the general population. However, the abnormalities may be caused by at least three separate things. First, the underlying abnormality that causes the mother's seizure disorder in the first place may also be responsible for the abnormality in the offspring; for example, a genetic biochemical condition such as phenylketonuria can cause seizures in the parent and possibly abnormalities in the child. Second, the seizures themselves may provoke fetal abnormalities. This is particularly so in the case of generalized tonic-clonic seizures because of the severe muscular contractions associated with them, which may damage the fetus, and because they may lead to decrease of oxygen in both mother and child. The third factor may be anticonvulsant drugs. If enough medication of almost any type is given to an animal, for example, the incidence of fetal abnormalities increases. Also, such things in common use as tobacco and alcohol are known to affect the fetus. These are things any pregnant woman should avoid.

The specific risk in taking anticonvulsants has been the subject of many studies. A recent, extensive study from Japan (Okuma et al., 1980) showed that the incidence of fetal malformations rose sharply when the number of drugs used for controlling seizures was increased. The risk was approximately 5 percent with one drug, such as trimethadione, phenobarbital, primidone, mephobarbital, pheneturide, or acetazolamide (but no risk with phenytoin, carbamazepine, or valproic acid). When two drugs were used, the incidence was 5.5 percent; when three, it was 11 percent; and when four drugs were used conjointly, the incidence was 23 percent. Clearly, if patients are taking anticonvulsants during pregnancy, the regime should be simplified as much as possible, preferably consisting of only one drug or no more than two to control the seizures. The use of multiple drugs may reflect the severity of the seizure disorder, and it is important that the seizures be controlled during pregnancy — especially generalized tonic-clonic ones; but it must also be noted that multiple drugs increase the risk to the fetus.

Other studies have described fetal abnormalities in connection with most of the anticonvulsant medications, including phenytoin, phenobarbital, and carbamazepine. There is no absolute proof that the medications alone are responsible for the abnormalities, however. One study showed that fetal abnormalities frequently occurred in relatives of the women who had seizures — relatives who were not taking medication and who did not themselves have seizures. Therefore, heredity does play a role, along with the seizures themselves, the underlying abnormalities, and the medications.

The major fetal abnormalities usually found are various types of heart defects, cleft palate, and mental retardation. The minor defects include abnormal fingernails or toenails. Bleeding problems may be present as a result of anticonvulsant drug effects on the liver of the fetus, and there seems to be a somewhat greater incidence of neurological disorders in babies whose mothers have epilepsy. Again, the causes are unclear.

At this time, physicians recommend that women with seizures who are taking anticonvulsant medication should be counseled before they become pregnant about the risk of fetal abnormalities. The medication should be continued at a level that will control the seizures in a reasonable way but also in a regime simplified enough to keep the risk of malformations at a minimum. Further study is needed to outline the exact nature and extent of fetal abnormalities, determine causes, and measure the risk.

If one identical twin has epilepsy, will the other also be expected eventually to have it?

It is difficult to obtain valid statistics on identical twins and epilepsy, primarily because of the limited numbers of such cases. Remember that only about one birth in every 400 produces identical twins, and only two to three children in 100 have epilepsy. However, the limited statistics on identical twins, who naturally have the same genetic makeup, show a high correspondence of seizure activity. If one identical twin has epilepsy, the risk is about 80 percent that the other twin will develop a seizure disorder. In the case of fraternal twins, however, the risk is about 7 percent that one fraternal twin will develop epilepsy if the other has the condition when neither parent has the disorder. If a parent has epilepsy, the risk of occurrence in the fraternal twin is about 13 percent, according to data from Metrakos and Metrakos (1969), who have done the primary studies in genetics of convulsive disorders.

Is epilepsy more likely when a child has cerebral palsy?

The incidence of epilepsy among children with cerebral palsy is markedly higher than among the normal population. The incidence ranges from 12 to 85 percent, depending upon the type of motor disorder. The risk of seizures varies in relation to the type of cerebral palsy. When the child has cerebral palsy of the athetoid type, epilepsy is infrequently seen. However, in cases of spastic cerebral palsy, seizures occur in from 66 to 85 percent of the cases.

Are there any famous young people with epilepsy?

Patty Wilson is an active teenager with epilepsy who lives near Los Angeles, California. She has complex partial seizures, which result in staring spells, confusion, and robotlike movements. At one time in her childhood Patty was uncoordinated and virtually friendless at school, but this is no longer true.

Patty's father is a distance runner, and she started running with him to develop strength, coordination, and a sense of accomplishment. Patty gradually increased the distance to marathon running with her father; later she joined the track team at her high school.

Patty gained international fame in the summer of 1977, when she began her marathon run from Los Angeles to Portland, Oregon, a distance of 1,310 miles. This was with the stated purpose of proving that epilepsy need not become one's handicap. As well as the long distance, Patty faced hardships of wind, rain, hecklers (though, thankfully, there were more who cheered), frequent blisters, pain, and a stress fracture of her leg soon after the start of the marathon. The last problem nearly aborted the marathon. Others would have stopped, but not Patty. She has also finished a three-month, 2,000-mile run from Minneapolis-St. Paul to the nation's capitol in Washington, D.C., to improve public understanding and raise money for research in epilepsy.

This now-famous girl is a good example of what a person with epilepsy can do with personal determination and purpose. Patty has become a symbol of personal triumph over a handicap when one has enough determination, combined with parental and peer support. Her story, told in a *Reader's Digest* article (April 1978) and in *Run Patty, Run*, by Sheila Cragg, is recommended reading for parents, teenagers, and siblings of a child with epilepsy.

Patty was selected only as an example. Actually, there are scores of famous young persons with epilepsy who have refused to let what some consider a handicap stand in their way. The list includes young people from nearly every walk of life, including television and movie stars, famous athletes, doctors, lawyers, a recent Miss America, and a United States congressman.

4

DIAGNOSIS AND TREATMENT

Where can we obtain medical consultation or locate a medical specialist?

The family physician is the best person to request consultation and will probably arrange at least one visit to a specialist.

If you are new to the area and have no family physician, contact the local medical society or neurology association for referral to a specialist or clinic in your area. Hospitals that specialize in seizure disorders are listed in the Epilepsy Foundation of America's *Guide to Epilepsy Services* (see Appendix A). We find this an essential reference, as it lists the available services in each state. It also indicates the fee basis, types of specialists available, and eligibility requirements. It is probably the most exhaustive reference source of the major clinical services available. You may also request a list of several appropriate specialists or a direct referral from a center for the developmentally disabled or Crippled Childrens' Service.

Once we have recognized and accepted that our child has seizures, why is the diagnosis so important?

The diagnosis is vitally important for several reasons:

1. To make certain the episodes experienced are epilepsy, rather than another condition.
2. To define the type of seizure, assess the severity, and chart the course of the condition. Different types of seizures respond to different types of anticonvulsants.
3. To seek the cause of the condition. In many cases, the cause remains unknown. However, it is important to know if the condition is one of a seizure disorder alone, or if the child has a specific syndrome of which seizures are only one aspect. For example, in tuberous sclerosis and in Sturge-Weber's disease, the seizures accompany body defects, skin disorders, or mental retardation. Parents need to know the basic elements of the diagnosis in order to know what to expect, and to prepare themselves for handling the situation.

We have just learned that our child has a seizure disorder. What should we do?

The first and most important thing to do is to calm yourself. Take time to adjust to this news. The information probably had an initial shock effect, and under these circumstances, people do not always make the best decisions. Many parents tend to overreact, expect the worst, and let their fears run rampant.

Since you now know that your child has a seizure disorder, the child is also undergoing diagnostic procedures and is under a physician's care. The major steps are already under way. Even though all the tests may not be completed or the anticonvulsant medication not yet fully regulated, remember how far ahead you are in having the disorder recognized.

Don't let the diagnosis frighten you. Your child is no different because of a diagnosis. It simply means that the doctors now know more about the child than before, and are in a position to begin the most important aspect — the treatment.

Your task as parents is to provide comfort and emotional support for your child. Begin to do some reading about seizure disorders. Listen closely to what your physician tells you and, above all, ask questions! Ask how you can help. Do not just assume you will be informed. Remember, you now have a partner in any decisions to be made — the physician or clinic conducting the evaluations. Parents do not need to carry the full burden alone.

What specifically will the doctor want to know about the seizures?

A precise and accurate description of the seizures is one of the most valuable aids to diagnosis, and the importance of the seizure history cannot be overemphasized. This is particularly useful for young children. The history may be critical in separating epileptic seizures from other conditions that resemble a seizure disorder. Many times the diagnostic staff members do not have an opportunity to observe the actual seizure and must rely on the report from the family or school. On repeat visits, the staff will rely on the report of any aspects of the seizure pattern that have changed.

Although members of the family are not always the best observers because of the emotion and excitement generated by a seizure, we have found that they can be trained to watch carefully if they know what questions might be asked, in relation to the seizure, during a detailed history of the seizures by the nurse or physician in diagnostic and follow-up visits.

The following questions are the most likely:

1. What was the person doing at the time of the seizure?
2. What took place before the seizure?
3. What was the exact time of day when the seizure occurred?
4. What called your attention to the seizure (a cry, fall, stare, arched back, etc.)?
5. How did the seizure develop (suddenly, gradually, in one part of the body, etc.)?
6. Did the person's body become rigid?
7. Were there jerks, twitches, or convulsions?
8. What part of the body moved first? Next?
9. Did the eyelids flutter or the eyes roll?
10. Did the person fall or change body position?

11. Did the skin show changes (become flushed, clammy, blue, etc.)?
12. Did the breathing change?
13. Did the person talk or perform any actions during the seizure?
14. Did the person become drowsy or sleep afterward?
15. Did the person urinate or have a bowel movement?
16. What was the length of the seizure?
17. Could you make contact with the person during the seizure? Was there a response?
18. What was the person's behavior like after the seizure (alert, drowsy, confused, remembering what happened, etc.)?
19. Did the person report any unusual feelings or sensations that happened before the seizure?
20. Is the person taking medication? When was the last dose?

Observers should try to recall the sequence of what happens to the person during the seizure and to estimate the time period as accurately as possible. Use a watch with a second hand if available. Any major variation from the typical pattern shown by the individual should be communicated to the physician prescribing the medication.

What type of evaluations should be expected?

When a person has a seizure or is thought to have a convulsive disorder, he should be evaluated by a physician or by a team in a clinic including a physician. The initial evaluation will include a careful and detailed history of the client and the family, including an accurate description of the seizure episodes. A general physical and neurological examination should be conducted. Laboratory studies of blood and urine will be made to detect any metabolic abnormalities such as low blood sugar or mineral deficiency. Major diagnostic tests will normally be ordered. In many cases, consultation with a neurologist will be sought for a more complete examination of the specific functions of the nervous system.

The major diagnostic tests routinely given are:

1. Electroencephalogram (EEG): a recording of the electrical activity of the brain
2. Computerized axial tomography (CAT scan): a picture of the internal structure of the brain compiled by density readings processed by a computer, showing any changes in density
3. Skull X rays: X rays of the bones of the skull that may reveal abnormalities, unknown fractures, or thickening of the bone. In certain conditions, areas of calcification may form within the brain and can be observed by this technique.

One or more of the following additional diagnostic tests may be needed in some cases, depending upon the findings of the neurological examination and medical history:

1. Nuclear brain scan: pictures of the pattern of transient absorption by the brain of certain nuclear isotopes injected into the bloodstream as it passes through the brain to assist in identifying areas of brain injury or tumor
2. Arteriogram: an X ray taken after a dye outlines the arteries and other blood vessels in the brain, showing any abnormalities
3. Pneumoencephalogram: X ray taken following injection of a small amount of air into the spinal canal, which then rises to the *ventricles* (spaces around and in the brain)
4. Lumbar puncture: removal of a small amount of spinal fluid to test for abnormalities
5. Special electroencephalogram: an EEG using specialized nasopharyngeal or sphenoidal electrodes or telemetry, or recorded under special conditions, such as sleep deprivation or drug-induced sleep.

Other studies may be conducted during the initial diagnostic phase, though sometimes they are delayed until later. A psychological examination may be necessary to determine the developmental level, especially with young children. This examination should include assessment of motor, language, and social skills of the child. The developmental examination may be conducted on children from ages six months to four years using tests such as the Gesell Developmental Scale, the Cattell Infant Intelligence Scale, the Bayley Scales of Infant Development, or the Denver Developmental Screening Test. The developmental examination may be periodically repeated to assess the rate of growth in each area.

Older children and adults should have an individual intelligence test such as the Wechsler Intelligence Scale or the Stanford-Binet Intelligence Scale. A specialized psychological assessment using the Halstead-Reitan Neuropsychological Test Battery may add information regarding the specific areas of functional deficit associated with a seizure disorder. Educational tests, including individual achievement tests, are important to assess the level of functioning in academic skills for school-age children. Special examinations may be conducted if the child has developed behavior or communication problems.

The EEG may be repeated periodically, and blood and urine samples required at regular intervals. When all of the studies have been completed, the physician or diagnostic team in the clinic (physician, consulting neurologist, clinical psychologist, educational specialist, and social worker or occupational therapist) will identify the type of convulsive disorder, determine the cause (if possible), and recommend treatments. Treatment with anticonvulsant medication is normally started as soon as possible and is given as a daily routine. Treatment may also involve a change in the home environment, placement in a specialized classroom, or counseling for emotional problems.

How can I be assured that my doctor knows of the latest techniques?

The professionals working with persons who have epilepsy can learn of new techniques from several sources. First, there are workshops and symposia sponsored by the International League Against Epilepsy, the American Epilepsy Society, the Western Institute on Epilepsy, and major university hospitals across the country. These are often cosponsored by local epilepsy societies. University medical centers also present post-graduate courses for physicians, EEG technicians, nurses, and other professionals. For example, one recent course known to the authors covered the following topics: a comprehensive review of the types of epilepsy and management, neonatal and atypical seizures, blood-level testing, new drugs, status epilepticus, and treatment of intractable seizures.

Many physicians also learn of new advances through medical videotapes, which include epilepsy, that are sent to local hospitals. A great number of physicians also subscribe to audio cassette tape services, which present the latest techniques of medical management to the practicing physician.

Another source of information is the Comprehensive Epilepsy Programs (see Chapter 8 and Appendix A), which demonstrate the newest advances in treatment and clinical investigation of epilepsy to physicians in the area. More technical information is available through the National Institute of Neurological and Communicative Disorders and Stroke (NINCDS) research papers and monographs. This agency also prepares *Epilepsy Abstracts,* which is a summary of all published articles relating to epilepsy, and sponsors EPILEPSY-LINE, which is a computer access to about 25,000 references and abstracts on epilepsy in medical libraries. The scientific journal exclusively concerned with epilepsy is *Epilepsia,* published by the American Epilepsy Society, which is an organization of professionals working in this specialty.

You may be assured that the latest information is available to your physician, who is undoubtedly already aware of such sources. Since you share a mutual concern, the doctor would probably appreciate any questions you might have as to whether he is utilizing these and/or other resources.

What is the EEG? How does it help determine whether one has epilepsy?

Since 1929, when Hans Berger first published his findings on brain rhythms, the EEG technique has advanced so rapidly that it is now considered one of the most important tests to help diagnose epilepsy.

By a technique of amplifying the brain waves some 100,000 times and writing them down mechanically on a moving paper roll, a permanent visual record is obtained. The EEG technique enables one to record the waves from several areas of the brain at the same time, and is thus vastly more complicated than the electrocardiogram (EKG), which records the electrical activity in the heart.

The electroencephalogram is actually a recording of the electrical activity of the brain. The recording is also commonly referred to as a "brain-wave tracing." Small disks (electrodes) are placed on the scalp with the help of special adhesive paste to hold them in place. Some units use tiny needles instead of disk electrodes. Wires run from the electrodes to the machine, which amplifies the tiny electrical discharges and records them on the moving paper with a series of pens. The final record is a series of wavy lines that show the voltage pattern of the nerve cells in various areas of the brain.

The process is entirely harmless, and the machine cannot injure the person in any way. There is no sensation with the disks, and the needle units cause only a small pinprick sensation. Generally, the person is sitting or lying down. He must be in a relaxed state, since other activity from movements in muscles of the forehead or scalp will also be recorded and will interfere with the tracing.

The EEG picks up the electrical impulses only from the surface of the brain. Internal and deep brain centers are not recorded by the "regular" EEG. Special depth electrodes may be used in a hospital setting to aid in the diagnosis of more complex cases. This involves inserting thin wires into the brain (a painless procedure) and recording the electrical discharges from the deep brain centers.

Special research EEG equipment may also be used in a hospital. A helmetlike EEG transmitter, worn on the head, sends the brain waves to a recording device in another room. The EEG and a videotape of the person may be made together, so that a recording of the abnormal discharges and the visual images of the seizures may be studied at the same time.

The EEG is not perfect, and a person with epilepsy may record normal brain waves. However, despite its limitations, the EEG can usually indicate whether a person has epilepsy and may suggest the type of condition present.

What are the limitations of the EEG?

As mentioned, the EEG is a valuable diagnostic tool that can determine the type of seizure by the form of the abnormal electrical discharge. In most cases, it will tell which part of the brain is sending the altered discharges, which are usually present even when the person is not having seizures.

Though the EEG is an extremely useful instrument, it does have its limitations, and parents must not expect too much from a reading. It is a laboratory test that must be interpreted and combined with other information for the fullest benefit.

The EEG cannot read a person's mind, record thoughts, or reveal personality or intelligence. It cannot specify how long a person will have seizures or when the next seizure may occur. It cannot indicate the cause of the seizures. It simply tells the status of the electrical activity on the surface of the brain at the time of the recording and indicates the particular area of the brain producing the abnormal discharge.

Does a "positive" or "abnormal" EEG reading mean a child has epilepsy?

Not necessarily. The EEG is one of the most helpful of all diagnostic tools, but it cannot tell everything. There may be abnormal activity in the brain that is not epileptic in nature. Furthermore, the EEG measures less than two thirds of the electrical activity in the brain, and usually does it in less than one half-hour. Remember that the electrical activity in the brain is constantly changing, and that the reading is merely a sample of the activity at the time of administration. As we mentioned, the EEG is an essential part of the diagnosis, but an abnormal reading does not necessarily establish the presence of epilepsy, nor does a normal EEG serve as a guarantee against its presence. Many people with epilepsy have normal EEGs between seizures.

Should the EEG be repeated at intervals to determine change?

The chief function of the EEG is as a guide in the initial diagnosis of a seizure disorder. It cannot be used alone to determine when medication should be discontinued or as a predictor of future seizures. For some persons the EEG remains abnormal even when the seizures are no longer present, and for others, the tracings may show as normal even when seizures continue. Some persons who have never had a seizure have abnormal EEG readings.

The relationship between the EEG and observed seizure activity is not very strong. Only in the case of petit-mal absence seizures do the seizure behavior and the EEG pattern match: the three-CPS spike-and-wave discharge pattern seen diffusely over the whole brain correlates well with the actual absence attack and decreased response time in the patient.

The physician will treat the observed seizures, not the EEG pattern; similarly, the psychologist or social worker treats the observed behavior. Family and professionals must deal with the whole person. To supplement information about the person during the course of treatment, additional EEGs may be recorded, but in general, the value of the EEG is in the initial diagnosis, not in determining ongoing treatment, except with petit-mal absence seizures.

What is the CAT scan?

The CAT (computerized axial tomography) scan is a relatively new tool in the diagnosis of neurological disorders. It shows the differences in densities from the skull to the brain to the spinal fluid inside the ventricles of the brain. Through the scan, a complete picture of the brain is made by compiling the density readings processed by a computer.

Many abnormalities of the brain have densities that differ from that of the normal brain tissue as well as from one another. This makes the CAT scan a relatively good tool in identifying such things as brain tumors, arteriovenous malformations, and cerebral vascular accidents (strokes). For example, a stroke may cause a swelling that decreases the density in that area of the brain; this will probably show up on the CAT scan — not always immediately, at the time of the stroke, but sometimes 7 to 10 days later, as the changes in the brain slowly take place.

A brain tumor can show up sometimes as an area of increased

density and sometimes as one of decreased density. One characteristic of a tumor is that when contrast material is injected into a person's vein and travels to the brain, the tumor will at times collect the contrast material, which will have an increased density compared with the rest of the brain. Without the contrast material, the tumor may be an area of decreased density. Different types of tumors will react differently and therefore will exhibit different patterns on the CAT scan. It is not possible, however, to tell the cell type of the tumor from the CAT scan alone, and additional tests will be needed to identify the type of tumor correctly. Arteriovenous malformations also may collect the intravenous contrast material and, like the tumors, will show up as areas of different density from their surroundings.

The CAT scan is revolutionary in medical diagnosis because it allows a great deal to be found out about the brain with very little risk to the patient. The amount of radiation required is less than that usually needed for a set of skull X-ray pictures. The original paper on the technique of CAT scanning was written by Dr. William Oldendorf, a neurologist, in 1961, but it took several years for the machine as well as the technique to be available commercially. It has enjoyed widespread use only since about 1974.

Is the X ray effective in the diagnosis of epilepsy?

In most persons with seizure disorders, plain X rays of the skull are no longer very helpful, unless there happens to be some calcification of the brain itself. This occurs very rarely in some types of parasitic diseases and in some tumors. The CAT scan has essentially replaced plain X rays.

There are, however, other tests, which, despite a certain degree of risk and discomfort, may be necessary to outline exactly what is happening inside the brain. One test is the cerebral angiogram: a contrast material is injected into the carotid artery, which goes directly into the brain. As the contrast material moves through the brain, a very rapid series of X-ray pictures is taken, from the front and the side, to outline the distribution of the blood vessels in the brain. Abnormalities will show up in this test that the CAT scan may not be able to discern. The risk in this procedure is much less than 1 percent, but physicians are reluctant to use it unless it will be constructive in indicating a change in a patient's treatment.

Another test is the pneumoencephalogram. This procedure is less risky than the angiogram when properly performed, but it is uncomfortable for the patient because it usually causes a severe headache. A lumbar puncture is performed, and either air or pure oxygen is injected into the space inside the spinal canal. This air then travels to the ventricles of the brain. The patient, who is seated in a special chair, is tilted this way and that to locate the air precisely while X-ray pictures are taken that will outline the structures of the brain in fine detail. Since the CAT scan is so precise in measuring fine differences in densities, the pneumoencephalogram is now seldom needed, but it can be helpful at times in outlining particular structures, especially those in the base of the brain and the brainstem. The physician must weigh the benefit of the information gained against the risk and discomfort of the procedure.

How is the Neuropsychological Test Battery used?

The Halstead-Reitan Neuropsychological Test Battery is comprised of a series of tests that assess the cognitive, perceptual, and motor skills of an individual. The battery is useful in determining the behavioral correlates of the clinical data in convulsive disorders.

Other psychological tests have been shown to offer clues as to whether a person might have epilepsy, but are of greater value in evaluating psychological disorders that may accompany epilepsy. Such evaluations are useful in designing a comprehensive treatment and rehabilitation plan for a child or adult.

How often does a person with epilepsy need to be reexamined?

Regular visits with the physician will be needed while attempting to bring the seizures under control and during any changes in medication. The physician will usually individualize the follow-up schedule depending upon the diagnosis, age of the person, and the necessity of monitoring medication effects. As children grow in size, and especially during adolescence when metabolism changes, the dosages of medication need to be adjusted regularly. Once the person is seizure-free, visits at least every six months are required while anticonvulsants are being taken.

The use of some drugs requires periodic blood analysis or urinalysis and tests of liver function, all of which require trips to the laboratory. Electroencephalograms may also be repeated periodically. For children having social or educational difficulties, periodic psychological or educational evaluations may be indicated.

Any major alterations in the nature or frequency of the seizure pattern warrants an immediate visit to the physician or clinic treating the person.

Is there a traditional treatment approach to epilepsy?

Yes. The basic treatment for seizure disorders is a combination of anticonvulsant medication, social and family adjustments, and counseling for teenagers and adults to help them deal with the problems related to epilepsy. This treatment plan is usually the "starting place" and is continued unless a variation is needed. Treatment must be directed toward the whole person, not just the seizures.

What is being done to prevent epilepsy?

Prevention of seizure disorders relies heavily on research into the basic cause of the disorder, since in so many cases of epilepsy the cause is unknown. Until a cause is isolated, prevention is an uncertain process. The importance of increased research, therefore, cannot be stressed enough. In areas where the cause is known, efforts are under way to assist in prevention.

Better prenatal and obstetric care is a basic approach to the prevention of epilepsy and other birth defects. The education of prospective parents regarding the importance of prenatal care, potential hazards of drugs and accidents, the need for good nutrition for prospective mothers, and the desirability of hospitalization for birth is vital in prevention. Reduction of infections such as German measles or meningitis is critical, especially during the first three months of pregnancy. The importance of obtaining childhood immunizations is essential, as serious early childhood diseases may lead to seizure disorders.

Avoidance or reduction of serious accidents to the head is also an essential preventive measure. Better public education to help reduce accidents is badly needed. The relaxation of mandatory motorcycle helmet laws, for example, has caused an increase in severe head injury. It has been estimated that between 20 and 45 percent of severe head injuries result in seizures, with serious automobile accidents considered the prime cause. The incidence of epilepsy could be markedly decreased with better child safety and careful driving. The campaign to mandate seat belts in autos is a positive step in this direction. The reduced 55-mile-per-hour speed limit has probably been the most effective measure of prevention of new cases of epilepsy by reducing the number and severity of head injuries from automobile accidents.

For those who already have epilepsy, it is usually possible to prevent continued seizures by careful adherence to medication and the avoidance of situations that produce stress.

What about surgical treatment for epilepsy?

The first successful surgery to treat a seizure disorder was performed in 1886 by the British neurologist Sir Victor Horsley. He removed a brain scar from a man of twenty-five who had suffered frequent focal attacks for ten years as a result of a head injury.

Surgical treatment for people with severe seizures has improved a good deal since that time and still is improving. Unfortunately, it is not effective in all patients. Because of its complexity, it should be done only in special centers by surgeons who have had a great deal of experience in performing it.

To be a candidate for surgery, the person should meet three criteria: First, he or she must have focal-onset seizures that start in an area of the brain that could be surgically removed with very little neurological deficit. For instance, if the temporal lobe is the locus of seizure onset, some of this lobe can be removed without seriously affecting the patient. If the seizures start in the speech area, however, removal of the seizure focus might lead to a very significant speech problem. The risk of that consequence would obviously outweigh the benefit of being seizure-free.

The second criterion is that the patient must be "medically refractory." This means that he must have tried all known anticonvulsants at good therapeutic levels, yet still continues to have seizures.

The third criterion is that the seizure disorder itself must seriously interfere with the patient's life. This is hard to document objectively; for the most part it must be left up to the patient to determine. If one feels that the disorder in all its ramifications interferes with one's life-style seriously enough to warrant the risk of surgery, this criterion is met.

Several surgical procedures have been developed. The most common, which is also the most successful, was developed primarily at the Montreal Neurologic Institute under Drs. Wilder Penfield and Herbert Jasper. In this procedure, the area of the brain in which the seizure disorder arises is removed. The most important presurgical problem to solve is to pinpoint that area. Most neurologists and neurosurgeons involved in this type of work feel that they should gather information from many sources. First, numerous EEGs are recorded to determine if the spike-and-wave discharge pattern that appears between seizures is diffusely spread over the brain or is concentrated in one area. Next, the patient is hospitalized so that long-term EEGs can record brain waves during actual seizures. This is done by taking surface recordings from the scalp as well as from the base of the brain by means of special electrodes inserted about an inch and a half inside the angles of the jaws. Since even these specialized EEGs record only from a small area of the brain, it may not be possible to localize the seizure area. Then at a later date electrodes may have to be implanted inside the brain at various strategic locations for further EEGs. In addition, the cerebral angiogram, pneumoencephalogram, and CAT scan will give useful information about any injuries to the brain or abnormalities. Very sophisticated psychological testing can also help to determine deficiencies in specific brain areas.

Another relatively new procedure, still at present in developmental stages, shows promise in determining what areas of the brain have decreased metabolism and therefore may possibly have been injured. A radioactive-labeled glucose (sugar) is injected into the brain and the actual metabolism in the brain cells is examined through a specialized CAT scan. It is interesting to note that during a seizure the seizure focus shows greatly increased metabolism, but in between seizures, the focus shows decreased metabolic activity.

When all the information from these various procedures is put together, the physicians can tell, usually, where the seizure discharge originates. If it is in an area that is not crucial to the patient's functioning, the brain area can then be removed, and the chances that the seizures will be controlled are very good. The scar on the brain resulting from the surgery does not seem to give rise to a new seizure focus as other injuries do.

For patients who are not candidates for this type of focal surgery, there are other procedures that may be helpful. The *corpus callosum* (the deep fibers that connect the two hemispheres of the brain) can be cut or sectioned, with some reported success. The technique is at this time experimental, however. Some physicians have implanted pacemakers in the *cerebellum* (the "little brain" behind the cerebrum), which is essentially responsible for balance. The pacemaker can stimulate the inhibitory electrical output of the cerebellum. When it was originally reported, this procedure seemed to have a significant rate of success in controlling intractable seizures. Within a year or two, however, most of the patients had just as many seizures as they had had before the cerebellar implant, and so most neurosurgeons have given it up as having no real long-term benefit.

In summary, surgery can be of great benefit to a selected person with seizures but only after he or she has tried all the anticonvulsive medications and has met all the criteria described above.

Is surgery too expensive to be feasible?

Recent reviews of the cost show that surgery for persons who qualify for it is indeed expensive. One medical college reports that the current average cost for simple procedures is $6,000, with an average charge of $19,000 for more complex operations. The costs include tests, hospitalization, the neurosurgeon, operating room, and post-operative visits.

The cost of the surgery, however, is more than offset by the benefits of added productivity in life. Many persons whose seizure disorders have seriously interfered with their life-styles and chances for employment can become seizure-free and employable after surgery. Since they can then pay taxes rather than receiving others' tax money, their improvement benefits the whole community. For those who qualify for surgery, the cost of it, therefore, is worthwhile not only in dollars-and-cents terms but also — and this is even more important — in terms of the improvement in the quality of their lives.

Should a physician be called when a person has a seizure?

Once a seizure has started it cannot be stopped, and no attempt should be made to do so. The seizure generally ends of its own accord and it is not necessary to call a physician. However, if the seizures become prolonged or occur in rapid succession, the doctor should be called. A report should be made of any person's having initial seizures and of any change in seizure pattern. It is not usually necessary to report to the physician each isolated seizure of a person receiving treatment.

What should a person do when he sees someone having a seizure?

Those persons associated with anyone who has epilepsy should be aware of the fact that seizures may occur, so that the event does not come as a surprise. Once one is aware of the possibility and a tonic-clonic seizure *does* occur, the following procedure is recommended:

1. Remain calm. Treat the incident in a matter-of-fact manner, and explain to others that the person is in no great or immediate danger to himself or to others, and that the seizure will most probably be over within a few minutes. As was mentioned, there is nothing that can be done to stop a

seizure once it has begun. If in a public place, simply request onlookers to leave.

2. Do not attempt to restrain the person's movements other than to prevent him from hurting himself. Loosen the clothing and be sure he is not near hot or sharp objects, such as a radiator, scissors, or the like. Clear the area around the person. Do not force anything between the teeth. Turn the person to one side so the saliva can flow from the mouth and the tongue can move forward and not block the windpipe. Place a pillow or folded coat under the head.

3. Stay with the person until the seizure is over and consciousness has returned. Offer reassurance if the seizure has left the person frightened or confused. Allow rest or sleep in a quiet place until the person is ready to assume normal activity.

4. It is usually not necessary to call a physician unless the attack lasts more than ten minutes or is followed by another major attack.

No first aid is necessary for absence seizures.

For partial complex seizures it is important not to attempt to restrain the person. Let the seizure take its course, but try to remove any harmful objects from the area. Again, offer reassurance if the person is frightened or remains confused. Stay with the person until he or she is fully capable of resuming activity.

Is there a risk of a person's swallowing his tongue during a seizure?

Of all the persisting rumors and misconceptions concerning epilepsy, this is perhaps the most dangerous. Actually, the person does not and cannot swallow his tongue during a seizure. During a generalized tonic-clonic seizure the muscles of the throat become so taut that the patient is unable to swallow. Placing a finger into the mouth of a person having a seizure or a solid object like a spoon or knife between the teeth is most dangerous and unnecessary. At the end of a generalized tonic-clonic seizure the muscles will relax and, if the person is lying on his back, the tongue can flop back and block the airway. To prevent this, turn the person onto his stomach or side.

What should one do when seizures occur during sleep?

Nocturnal epilepsy presents some specific problems not present in other seizure patterns, inasmuch as the person with this condition usually has seizures *only* during sleep. Sleep progresses through several distinct stages and degrees of depth with accompanying changes in electrical activity. Seizures may occur during any of the stages of sleep, frequently when the patient is just going to sleep or just waking up. They can, however, happen at any time during sleep. It is hypothesized that sleep brings on or allows the release of abnormal electrical discharges in susceptible individuals. Persons prone to sleep seizures should avoid taking naps during the day and make adequate allowance for a full sleep period at night. Seizures at night actually cause fewer restrictions on a person's life than those occurring during the day.

A number of parents seen by the authors have been concerned about their child's nighttime seizures. The situation is frequently anxiety-provoking, and the parents often feel they must either watch the child at sleep or sleep with the child in order to be available to assist in case of a seizure. This is rarely warranted. The child experiencing seizures at night returns to sleep, and the parents may not even be aware of the event. Parents anxious about the situation often become tired and deprived of sleep, having been up during the day and part of the night on a regular basis.

In these cases, we have suggested installation of an inexpensive intercom between the parents' room and the child's bedroom. This simple unit may be set on "monitor" in the child's room at night and will awaken the parents when they hear the sounds of seizures. Most parents easily become attuned, if they are not already, to the sounds. We have found parents are able to get more rest and can easily learn to adjust to the device, waking up immediately when a seizure occurs. Furthermore, it lets the child be considered more "normal" than if he were watched or slept with at night. Simple intercoms may be purchased at local department stores or radio supply stores.

What should be done in the event of status epilepticus?

Status epilepticus is a serious medical emergency that requires immediate emergency hospital treatment. If the person has a series of generalized tonic-clonic attacks without regaining consciousness, the physician should be called immediately, and the person transported by ambulance to the nearest emergency room. Oxygen is necessary if cyanosis is present. Intravenous diazepam (Valium) is often given to stop the seizures immediately. Usually, however, this is not effective in long-term control of status epilepticus; the person may start having seizures again within half an hour. Additional drugs may be needed to control the seizures fully.

At a recent international symposium on status epilepticus, the consensus was that in adults intravenous diazepam should be followed by intravenous phenytoin (Dilantin), given no faster than 50 mgs per minute under careful monitoring. This was considered the most effective means of controlling status with the fewest side effects (such as sedation or respiratory depression). A consensus for the treatment of status epilepticus in children was not reached; some physicians preferred intravenous phenobarbital, others, intravenous phenytoin.

Treatment consists of establishing the proper balance or restoration of the anticonvulsant medication. Untreated, status epilepticus can result in irreversible brain damage as a result of prolonged hypoxia and even death.

When does a person with epilepsy need to be hospitalized?

The only situation requiring emergency hospitalization is status epilepticus. The person in this situation must be rushed to the nearest hospital emergency room as soon as possible, where prompt treatment to stop the seizures can be given. All other conditions involving hospitalization for epilepsy are at the option of the physician, and a parent does not need to be concerned about whether a child should be hospitalized.

Occasionally, it is necessary for some children to be placed in a hospital for the purposes of diagnostic procedures and observation of the seizures. This may be needed for a child with extended, uncontrolled seizures, or when the seizures are of an unusual type. Many physicians also request hospitalization during the initial stages of establishing a ketogenic diet (see page 77).

Most diagnostic procedures for epilepsy, however, are done in a physician's office or clinic, and except for status epilepticus there is no need to rush the patient to a hospital.

What should I do after my child has had a seizure?

The best move is simply to let the child rest or sleep as he wishes. Avoid excitement on *your* part, which can only add to feelings of embarrassment.

Are there methods of seizure control other than medication?

Yes, although they are still largely in experimental stages. Several research studies have been made of the use of biofeedback for management of epileptic seizures. Barry Sterman, Ph.D., originally suggested this use after his experiments with cats indicated that a resistance to seizure development could be brought about by inducing a certain type of brain-wave rhythm in the sensory-motor cortex. One recent study is that made by Lubar and Bahler (1976) of severely afflicted patients who were trained in self-control of their EEG rhythms solely by the use of biofeedback. The patients selected had epilepsy that could not be adequately controlled medically, resulting in frequent, uncontrolled seizures. With the use of specialized equipment in treatment sessions, the patients learned to inhibit specific seizure discharges. Once they had learned this control, usually they no longer needed the biofeedback equipment.

Following the biofeedback training, all of the patients in this study showed varying degrees of improvement. Some improved dramatically, with a marked decrease in seizure intensity; some were able to block the seizures totally.

Other researchers have not been able to attain such felicitous results. Biofeedback at present is still experimental and is available only at some research hospitals. Certainly it does decrease seizure frequency in some people, but we must stress that most of them are still on anticonvulsant medication and that biofeedback serves merely as an adjunct to, not a primary method for, seizure control.

Some people have invented their own "biofeedback" to prevent or abort a seizure. For instance, an individual whose seizures start with a focal area of tingling or numbness in one hand may have found that rubbing the hand vigorously can interfere with the seizure discharge and avert a full-blown seizure. Others have found that if they concentrate hard on something they may abort the seizure. It has been known for a long time that activity, such as working at a paid job or pursuing a much-enjoyed hobby, will lower the frequency of seizures.

A revolutionary treatment using behavior modification has been successfully used by Dr. Joseph Cautela and others at Boston College (1975). Though this method is still experimental and has had limited success, it has frequently been able to contain seizures in some children for whom medication has not been effective. The technique is a simple one in which the child learns both to reach a state of complete relaxation and to tighten his muscles when needed. When a seizure is averted, the child is given praise and/or other rewards or "reinforcement." When a seizure does occur, the behavior is not reinforced but is virtually ignored.

In keeping with the principles of behavior modification, the "undesirable" behavior (seizure) is not reinforced by attention, and the "desirable" behavior (avoiding a seizure) *is* reinforced by attention. The preliminary work of teaching the child the technique of thinking of pleasant, relaxing things when the aura begins is the most difficult part of this method, but various authorities consider behavior modification to be a viable alternative for cases for which there seems to be no other effective treatment.

Several new instruments are in the process of development, including an EEG warning device worn by the person, which signals the onset of a seizure and allows precautionary measures to be taken. Unfortunately, further research on this project has been delayed for lack of funding.

What is the ketogenic diet?

The ketogenic diet is one means of controlling seizures through diet. The diet is used primarily in persons for whom drug therapy has not been effective and is based on the fact that fasting has long been used as a means of seizure control. Indeed, during the days before anticonvulsants, there were few other alternatives.

The ketogenic diet attempts to stimulate the metabolic activity of the body during the early stages of fasting. Though the exact mechanism of the process is still a mystery, it has been used with some limited success. The diet itself is made up primarily of foods with a high fat and low carbohydrate content.

There are several disadvantages to the ketogenic diet. It is not pleasing to the taste, and the person often feels inclined to "cheat" occasionally after a few days, which means that the balance needs to be reestablished. It is especially difficult for parents to prepare the diet without errors. The diet also requires a daily urine test to guarantee the chemical changes. Some physicians limit the treatment to young children, whose diet is more easily totally controlled. Still other physicians use the initial treatment only in hospitals, with careful instructions to the parents on its continuance after the child is returned home. The ketogenic diet is used primarily as an alternative, when anticonvulsants have not been successful.

A more palatable diet can be given in some instances to children with myoclonic seizures, using median-chain triglycerides (MCT oil). Parents should consult a dietitian in preparing this or a ketogenic diet.

Can vitamins or minerals have a favorable effect on epilepsy?

This often-asked question is too complex for a simple yes or no, but must be answered for specific cases by an informed physician. There have been rare cases in which insufficient vitamin B_6 or magnesium has led to seizures. In other cases in which the child's metabolism may not be normal, the child's condition may have in turn created the vitamin or mineral deficiency.

A number of studies have explored the use of vitamins for seizure control, with the results showing little, if any, effect and in some cases even reporting increased seizures.

Recently, several articles on megavitamin therapy (vitamins given in massive doses) have been published in popular magazines. They

DIAGNOSIS AND TREATMENT / 79

suggest that megavitamins can be of assistance in a number of handicapping conditions. At present, there is no conclusive evidence that megavitamins have any anticonvulsive effect, and by no means should they be given unless prescribed by a physician.

Overall, unless the child is on the prescribed ketogenic diet for seizure control, no special foods or diet are needed. If the child does not eat well, the physician may want to add a simple vitamin supplement to the daily intake.

Can epilepsy be "cured"?

Technically, the condition cannot be cured except in a very few cases in which brain surgery can be performed. In most people, however, the seizures can be controlled or arrested. It has been estimated that in about 80 percent of the cases, it is possible to achieve either total or nearly complete seizure control. In these cases, the term "seizure arrest" would be more appropriate than "cure." In many cases, an individual will be seizure-free for years after anticonvulsant medication is discontinued. In this sense the person may be considered to have attained recovery or at least extended remission.

Can the adult with epilepsy drink alcohol?

There is no evidence at present to indicate that alcoholic beverages have a *direct* relationship with seizures. Indeed, alcohol is a mild anticonvulsant since it has a sedative effect. Most physicians, however, strongly advise moderation in the consumption of alcohol for two reasons. First, alcohol may react unfavorably with the anticonvulsant drug or drugs the person is taking. Since they both depress the central nervous system, the combination will produce drunkenness more quickly than alcohol would alone. It is important to continue taking the anticonvulsants, so the person with epilepsy must be particularly aware of the amount he can drink safely.

The second reason for moderation is that the excessive use of alcohol will often precipitate seizures. In general, a person who drinks enough to become drunk greatly increases the risk of having a seizure 12 to 24 hours afterward. Thus many neurologists advise their patients not to drink at all. Most, however, will suggest a very moderate alcohol intake — a glass of wine or one drink at dinnertime — if the patient desires it.

What about the use of marijuana (pot)?

Much research still needs to be done on the relationship between marijuana and seizures. Like alcohol, marijuana is a mild anticonvulsant; but also like alcohol, abrupt cessation in the use of marijuana after a period of excessive use may increase the frequency of seizures. All the answers are by no means in on this question.

Does my child need a protective helmet?

Some children and a few adults with severe seizures or with repeated daily seizures often tend to injure themselves during a fall. Such individuals can be assisted by routinely wearing a protective padded helmet. The helmet itself does not interfere with normal activities, but in case of a seizure does protect the person from a bruise or laceration to the head.

One should obtain a helmet that is lightweight and comfortable. It is not necessary to have a dome helmet (as in football gear), which is cumbersome, unsightly, and heavy. We have found a lightweight plastic or vinyl padded model (similar to those worn by bicycle riders or boxers during workouts) to serve very well. It may be secured by a chin strap or chin pad. These helmets may be purchased at any hospital equipment and medical supply store. If you cannot find one, write Danmar Corporation, 2390 Winewood, Ann Arbor, Michigan 48103.

Some parents do not want their child to appear "different" by wearing a helmet. Our experience has been that the children accept the helmet readily, but the parents have difficulty with the idea. The child easily becomes accustomed to putting it on especially if it is introduced as his "play helmet" or his very own football helmet and is associated with pleasant activities. The parent should put it on the child in the same emotional tone used to tell the child that he needs a coat before going outside in cold weather. It is far kinder to protect the child from serious injury than to assume the child will resist the helmet.

We have seen a few examples of a new, plastic protective "wig," used primarily by girls, which often resembles a standard wig worn regularly by women. One mother of our acquaintance routinely puts her own wig on when she asks her daughter to put on her "wig."

A new lightweight, polyethylene foam protective helmet is currently under development by the Rehabilitation Medicine Research and Training Center at George Washington University. The foam protector is custom-made to fit as a band around the skull and can be worn unobtrusively under a wig or hat. It is made from materials developed for their light weight and shock-absorbent properties by the National Aeronautics and Space Administration. The headgear is undergoing further tests and is as yet not commercially available.

What about residential or hospital facilities?

Most persons with seizures can and should live in their own communities. There are circumstances, however, where residential care is beneficial and preferable. Placement in a hospital is sometimes needed to achieve good seizure control in complex cases. For persons with multiple handicaps, including seizures, residential placements permit the various medical rehabilitation treatment services to be given in one location and as a coordinated plan, which is beyond the ability of the local community to provide.

Management of severe and uncontrolled seizures can also be physically and emotionally draining to a family, and there are times when a hospital with an experienced staff can and should (and in some cases *must)* relieve the strain. Occasionally, young adults with only partial control of seizures may also benefit from foster-placement living to gain greater independence from the family. Residential schools may be able to provide the specific education or vocational training that may not be available in the local community.

There is a wide range of facilities available in some areas, few or no resources in others. The types of facilities include community foster homes, convalescent hospital or intermediate care facilities, private and public institutions for the mentally ill and/or the developmentally disabled. Generally, these institutions do not exist solely for persons with seizures, but they may accept persons with seizure disorders as well as other handicaps. Significant improvements have occurred in public institutions and in convalescent hospitals in recent years. Foster homes can provide supervised group living arrangements. In some areas, programs are available for supervised apartment living, which is a relatively new and growing concept. This offers semi-independent living for young adults who need some supervision in residential living and assistance in money management or personal skills, but who also need feelings of independence.

The decision for residential placement must, of course, be carefully considered. Any institutional facility should have an individualized treatment plan and adequate services to provide the level of care needed.

You will probably need guidance in selecting an appropriate facility from a mental health center, an epilepsy clinic, your physician, or the local epilepsy chapter. You should also check the directories listed in Appendix A of this book as a source guide.

I have heard epilepsy referred to as the "most expensive" of the disorders. Is this true?

Epilepsy is by far the most expensive of all neurological disorders. In 1975, the estimated cost of epilepsy in the United States was more than three billion dollars. The Epilepsy Foundation of America now estimates that the annual cost in the United States alone is $4,370,000,000! The figures for costs to individuals with epilepsy are equally staggering. The average annual cost for medical treatment is $250 per person, plus an average annual expenditure of $213 for anticonvulsants. In addition, there is a myriad of hidden costs to the person with epilepsy; for example, the average weekly salary of employed persons with epilepsy is nearly $40 per week less than that of employed persons who do not have epilepsy. Furthermore, the unemployment rate of persons with epilepsy is double that of the national rate.

The following 1975 statistics were reported by the Commission for the Control of Epilepsy and Its Consequences in Volume I of its Plan for Nationwide Action on Epilepsy, released in late 1977 (the figures reported refer to persons with epilepsy):

1. The cost of unemployment reached more than one billion dollars.
2. Underemployment because these persons often must take unskilled or semiskilled positions totaled an estimated salary loss of $517,000,000.
3. Excess mortality cost $435,000,000.
4. Costs of treatment reached nearly $333,000,000.
5. Institutional and residential care cost more than one and a quarter billion dollars.
6. Cost of drugs for seizure control is estimated at $110,000,000.
7. Vocational rehabilitation cost $13,000,000.
8. Special education cost $64,000,000.
9. Research cost $38,000,000.

Though the primary concern in forming the commission to develop a Nationwide Plan was humanitarian rather than economic, it can readily be seen that in addition to saving and changing human lives, the control of epilepsy would also save a great deal of money. Epilepsy is a terribly expensive disorder — in human as well as economic costs.

5

ANTICONVULSANTS

What guidelines does the physician use in drug therapy?

For a person with a seizure disorder, the physician will try to find a treatment that has the best therapeutic effect with the fewest side effects; in other words, one that controls seizures without causing any new problems. In general, it is usually better to use one drug rather than two, but for some patients a combination of drugs will be more effective than a single one: if one drug alone will not control the seizures, then two may be necessary, but rarely more than two at one time. The physician will start the patient on the drug of choice for the particular type of seizure. The dosage is determined initially by the age and weight of the person; it will gradually be increased to the most effective level or point of tolerance. During the initial period, the physician will need a report on the number of seizures that occur and any change in the seizure pattern. After the higher limits of the drug have been reached, the doctor may add or substitute a second drug if the seizures are not yet controlled.

Once the drug or combination of drugs produces the best level of control without any side effects, this level must be maintained by regular use of the medication. Here the cooperation of family members and school personnel is vital, since they are in far better positions than the physician is to observe periodic changes in behavior or seizure frequency.

As a guide in drug therapy, the physician will periodically take blood samples to determine the *serum level* — the proportion in the blood — of the various drugs used. A great deal of study has been done as to the most effective level that will control seizures with each of the drugs individually. In addition, the level at which a drug will cause toxic side effects in most individuals has been determined. Therefore, the physician will try to get a serum level in the "therapeutic range." This term is used as a sort of catch-all to mean the serum level at which a person who has seizures will have them controlled if they are going to be controlled on that particular medication. The therapeutic range may vary from person to person, and not everyone will have his or her seizures controlled by a drug within the therapeutic range. Levels in the *toxic range* mean that there will be deleterious side effects, such as drowsiness or sedation or problems with balance or other conditions.

A physician, however, doesn't treat ranges or levels in patients; he treats the patient. The aim of seizure control without side effects may be achieved at different serum levels for different persons, and so the levels must not serve as rigid guides.

In some persons increased seizure frequency has been noted when they are given too much medication and are actually in the toxic range. Most physicians are aware of this and try to guard against it.

What drugs are used to control epilepsy?

A number of anticonvulsant medications are effective for control of various types of seizures. Although epileptologists (neurologists who specialize in the treatment of seizure disorders) differ in their opinions as to those drugs which are the most effective for particular seizure types, there are some general drugs of choice. The six major ones are listed in the chart, with their approximate therapeutic levels, toxic levels, half-lives, and the time it takes for the drug to reach a therapeutic level if the usual dose is given.

Following is a description of the major drugs, as well as some of the second-line drugs. They are listed by generic name, with the trade name given in parentheses.

THERAPEUTIC RANGES OF VARIOUS ANTICONVULSANTS

DRUG	THERAPEUTIC LEVEL (IN MICROGRAMS PER MILLILITER)	TOXIC LEVEL (EQUAL TO OR GREATER THAN)	APPROXIMATE HALF-LIFE[a] (IN HOURS)	TIME TO REACH STEADY STATE[b] (IN DAYS)
carbamazepine	8–12	12	6–8	3–4
phenytoin	10–20	30	20–24	7–10
phenobarbital	20–40	50	55–140	21
primidone[c]	6–10	12	6–8	3–4
valproic acid	50–100	120	8–12	4–5
ethosuximide	50–100	120	50–60[d]	10–15

[a]This refers to the time it takes for the serum level to reach one half its present value if no further dose of the drug is taken; i.e., the time it takes to clear one half the drug from the body.

[b]This is the time it takes for the serum level to reach a steady or level state if normal doses of the drug are taken daily.

[c]Primidone is also converted to phenobarbital, which has a very long half-life.

[d]Half-life in children is about 30 hours.

MAJOR DRUGS

Carbamazepine (Tegretol). This is a major drug for control of focal-onset, secondarily generalized seizures such as partial simple, partial complex (psychomotor or temporal lobe), and secondarily generalized tonic-clonic seizures, and also for generalized-onset tonic-clonic seizures. Many epileptologists consider it the drug of choice for this type of seizure. When this drug was first used, blood abnormalities, such as bone-marrow suppression and aplastic anemia, were discussed intensely by professionals. Anthony Pisciotta, M.D., made a thorough review of the world literature concerning carbamazepine's side effects, which was published in *Advances in Neurology* in 1975. He could find only three cases of aplastic anemia, a condition in which the bone marrow shuts down entirely and the risk of death is high, probably directly related to carbamazepine. The rest of the reported cases of aplastic anemia were felt possibly to be associated with the drug, but the connection was by no means proved. Hundreds of thousands of patients have taken the drug safely.

Usually carbamazepine should be started at a very low dosage and gradually increased, because drowsiness is a noticeable side effect at first. Once the patient is accustomed to the drug, this effect becomes minimal. At the beginning of use of carbamazepine, the patient must have complete blood counts and liver enzyme tests taken at biweekly intervals; later, these tests can be performed every one to two months. The tests are to ensure that no serious side effects are occurring. At high levels, the medication can cause drowsiness, dizziness, and balance problems.

Phenytoin (Dilantin). This major drug of choice has been used since 1938 for focal-onset seizures, secondarily generalized tonic-clonic seizures, and generalized-onset tonic-clonic seizures. Many neurologists consider it the first drug of choice for these types. In the therapeutic range it does not usually cause excessive drowsiness. It has been reported to increase body and facial hair growth and growth of gum tissue *(gingival hyperplasia).* Good dental hygiene can help to prevent the growth of gum tissue by keeping down the concentration of phenytoin in the saliva. One should brush the teeth at least twice a day and rinse the mouth out with water in between times, particularly at lunchtime. At toxic doses, the patient can have a problem with balance and may feel drowsy. Often, the first sign of toxicity is double vision. These side effects can be reduced by decreasing the dosage.

Phenobarbital. This is the oldest anticonvulsant in consistent use today, having been introduced in 1912. It is effective for focal-onset as well as generalized tonic-clonic seizures. It is relatively inexpensive compared with other drugs. However, phenobarbital does cause more drowsiness for the same therapeutic benefit than do phenytoin and carbamazepine. If the drug is at toxic levels, the patient will be significantly slowed down and drowsy, and may have a balance problem. This drug can aggravate hyperactivity in some children with the hyperactive syndrome.

Primidone (Mysoline). Introduced in 1953, this drug is effective against generalized tonic-clonic and focal-onset seizures. Primidone, an anticonvulsant in its own right, is converted to phenobarbital and PEMA (phenylethylmalonamide), both of which have anticonvulsant effects. Although the drug is very effective in treating seizures, the side effects are usually greater than those seen with the first three drugs. Particularly in teenagers, behavioral problems may become much worse, even when the drug is in therapeutic ranges; when it is gradually discontinued, the behavior improves.

Because primidone when first used causes severe drowsiness and dizziness, it can never be started at the usual therapeutic dosage. It is begun at a dosage of one eighth or one fourth of a tablet given at nighttime and then very slowly and gradually increased to the therapeutic range. In the toxic range the drowsiness becomes pronounced, and a problem with balance may develop.

Valproic acid (Depakene). This is a major drug for treatment of petit-mal absence seizures as well as myoclonic and atonic seizures. The sedative side effects of valproic acid are far less severe than those of any anticonvulsant we have studied. Stomach irritation and indigestion can appear when a patient first starts using valproic acid, but if the dosage is low, the medication is taken with meals, and the amount is very gradually increased, almost everyone can tolerate the gastrointestinal effects, which eventually disappear. After one has become accustomed to the drug, one can often take it apart from meals without any significant effect on the stomach.

Liver toxicity and bleeding problems have also been reported with this drug. Because of its effect on the blood platelets, it may give rise to easy bruising (an effect also sometimes noted with aspirin). Patient and physician both should be aware of these side effects, particularly if surgery were to be necessary, though they are generally not significant. Approximately one or two weeks after the drug is started, and every one to two months thereafter, liver enzyme tests and blood counts should be obtained. Other side effects include thinning of the hair, which usually reverses itself; tremor, which is dose-related and is corrected by lowering the dose; and coma. Coma is a very rare problem usually seen in patients already on phenobarbital, and may be related to an increase in the ammonia level in the blood. Petit-mal status has been reported when valproic acid is used in conjunction with clonazepam.

One of the major advantages of valproic acid is that it is also effective against generalized tonic-clonic seizures, although less so than the other major anticonvulsants. Since about 40 to 50 percent of the people with absence seizures may at some time experience generalized tonic-clonic seizures, this drug can be used as the single drug for seizure control in some patients.

Ethosuximide (Zarontin). This is another major drug for treatment of absence seizures that also has some effect on myoclonic and atonic seizures. This drug may cause some stomach irritation when it is first used, and it must be begun gradually. Though it is very effective for absence seizures, at high dosages it will cause restlessness and drowsiness. It is not effective for generalized tonic-clonic seizures, so that if a patient has both types, he must use a second drug (such as phenytoin or carbamazepine) to control the generalized tonic-clonic ones.

SECOND-LINE DRUGS

Mephenytoin (Mesantoin). This is a second-line drug, similar to phenytoin, for treatment of generalized tonic-clonic and focal-onset seizures. The advantages of mephenytoin are that it is very effective and that it does not cause excessive hair growth or gingival hyperplasia, as does phenytoin. It has the disadvantages of causing some problems with the bone marrow in forming red blood cells and possibly aplastic anemia, which carries a risk of death if not handled properly. Though these effects are rare, the patient must be carefully monitored for them. At high levels, the drug can cause sedation and ataxia.

Mephobarbital (Mebaral). Directly converted to phenobarbital, this drug is essentially another form of that drug.

Ethotoin (Peganone). Another drug structurally similar to phenytoin, this is minimally toxic but also minimally effective. It is sometimes used for generalized tonic-clonic and focal-onset seizures when other medications have not proved useful. Gum growth and hair growth are seldom seen with ethotoin.

Acetazolamide (Diamox). This is a second-line drug commonly used as a diuretic that also has a mild anticonvulsant effect. It is generally used as an adjunct to other drugs, such as phenytoin or carbamazepine, particularly in female patients whose seizures are most often associated with the menstrual period.

Diazepam (Valium). This tranquilizer is occasionally used as an adjunct for controlling myoclonic and atonic seizures, in particular. It does cause sedation. It is an excellent drug given intravenously for initial control of status epilepticus, but another drug must be used for long-term control.

Clonazepam (Clonopin). Closely related to diazepam, this drug is effective for myoclonic and atonic seizures, but its sedative effect is fairly significant. Hair loss is another reported side effect, and at high levels, ataxia or balance problems may appear. Clonazepam should be used warily or not at all with valproic acid because of the risk of petit-mal status. In addition, clinical experience has indicated that the initial effectiveness of clonazepam for absence, myoclonic, and atonic seizures can wear off after one or two months — a development not common among other anticonvulsants.

Methsuximide (Celontin). This drug is structurally related to ethosuximide. It is effective against absence seizures, myoclonic jerks, and atonic seizures. At high levels, it can cause irritability and drowsiness. There have been some reports that it is also effective against generalized tonic-clonic seizures, which is not true for ethosuximide.

Dextroamphetamine (Dexedrine). This drug has a mild anticonvulsant action and is used to counteract the drowsiness resulting from one of the more sedating medications, such as phenobarbital or primidone. If one is dealing with the sedative side effects of another medication, however, it is better to adjust that medication rather than add yet another one to stimulate the patient. It is similar to whipping a tired horse and for the most part is not good treatment. Amphetamines such as dextroamphetamine do have some mild anticonvulsant properties and can occasionally be used for seizure control.

Corticotropin (ACTH). ACTH is a pituitary hormone that has been effective in treating myoclonic epilepsy, particularly the infantile spasms and hypsarrhythmia of the Lennox-Gestaut-West syndrome. *Hypsarrhythmia* is the term given to an abnormality in an infant that shows on the EEG as diffuse, slow brain waves with multiple focal spike-and-wave discharges. The condition is usually associated with a severe neurological problem and mental retardation. Treatment with ACTH has been effective.

SUMMARY

In general, the anticonvulsant used will depend on the type of seizure. For absence or myoclonic seizures, the first drug of choice is valproic acid or ethosuximide. For focal-onset seizures, including partial simple and partial complex (temporal lobe) seizures, and for generalized tonic-clonic seizures, the drugs of choice are carbamazepine, phenytoin, phenobarbital, and primidone.

A good deal of trial and error is involved in selecting the most appropriate medical regime for a particular patient, always with the aim of seizure control and the fewest side effects. The patient must be willing to work closely with the physician and try different types of anticonvulsants at good therapeutic levels in order to find that drug or combination of drugs which will be most effective.

I understand valproic acid is new in the United States. Can you tell me more about it?

Valproic acid was released for limited use in the United States by the Food and Drug Administration in early 1978, after a lengthy review. The drug itself, however, is not new, having been discovered in 1881. It was not until 1963 that its seizure control properties were discovered almost by accident. In 1967, valproic acid was licensed as an anticonvulsant in France and was used for another ten years in Europe and throughout much of the world before its introduction into this country. Although there were a number of studies and clinical reports on the drug, the FDA rules require that at least two scientifically controlled "double-blind" studies attest to a drug's efficacy. The Suzuki study, done in Japan in 1974, demonstrated improvement in children with absence epilepsy who had been treated unsuccessfully with other drugs. In 1978, a second double-blind study was conducted at the University of Virginia. The results confirmed the drug's usefulness in the reduction of absence seizures.

Delays from the FDA led to the setting up of an independent review committee by the Epilepsy Foundation of America, which, along with consumer pressure, was influential in winning the final approval for the drug. The FDA currently authorizes its limited use for simple or complex absence seizures or in combination with other drugs for persons who have multiple seizure types, including absence seizures. There is evidence that valproic acid is useful in major motor, focal, and myoclonic seizures, but it is not yet authorized for use in these conditions unless absence seizures are also present.

The chemistry of the anticonvulsant effect of valproic acid has not yet been clearly established. Some researchers have suggested that it increases the action of gamma-aminobutric acid (GABA), an inhibitory substance in the brain that helps control seizures. Valproic acid is a simple fatty acid and as such is chemically unrelated to other types of anticonvulsants in present use. It can be combined with other drugs, but must be given carefully, if at all, with clonazepam. It can also interact with phenobarbital, aggravating drowsiness, ataxia, and disorientation.

In general, however, this drug shows promise of improved seizure control, especially for absence seizures.

What are the most important things to know about side effects?

All drugs have effects in the body — some useful, some undesirable. The undesirable ones are known as "side effects." Side effects can occur with both prescription and nonprescription (over-the-counter) drugs and may increase when several drugs interact. The physician must be aware of all drugs a patient is regularly taking when an anticonvulsant is prescribed.

A person may be allergic to any given medication. The allergy may appear in many different ways, from a skin rash to a decrease in bone-marrow production of red and white blood cells. The latter effect can be very serious; moreover, it is idiosyncratic, meaning that it cannot be predicted from one patient to another. Fortunately, it is fairly rare. If a person develops a skin rash shortly after starting a medication, it must be assumed that he is allergic to it and it should not be given for seizure control.

Other side effects are dose-related, not allergic, and may appear in almost anyone if the anticonvulsant level is in the toxic range. They include fatigue, lack of interest, transient sleepiness, severe lethargy, ataxia (problems with balance), blurred vision, double vision, slurred speech, or clumsy movements. Such effects can be lessened by decreasing the amount of medication. Since seizures rarely are better controlled and can even be made worse when a drug is in the toxic range, it does no good to push the medication level above the therapeutic range, particularly when the side effects are present. Nor should you change the medication on your own even if side effects are present. Contact the physician and report the effects observed.

Why is one requested to continue having blood tests when one no longer has seizures?

Routine laboratory tests are required when one has been taking certain anticonvulsants. These tests can detect situations that could perhaps cause serious problems. Blood tests determine the therapeutic serum level of the medication. This information helps in adjusting dosages to provide maximum control with minimum side effects. With certain drugs, too, blood tests may be necessary even when the patient's seizures are completely controlled, to keep watch over effects of the medication on liver enzymes and blood counts.

Why do the drugs seem to make my child sluggish?

Drowsiness or sluggishness is a frequent side effect of a new drug until the medication level is established. Also, excessive medication can produce drowsiness and physical as well as mental lethargy. Typically, once the level is adjusted these symptoms disappear.

In some cases, however, the amount of medication necessary to stop the seizures also produces the undesirable side effects mentioned above. In this instance, one has to consider the alternatives of having elimination of seizures in connection with sluggishness *or* a more alert but seizure-prone child. Although the latter might seem the better alternative, the choice should be determined with your physician. When complete seizure control is not possible, the task becomes one of achieving the best balance between seizure frequency and the side effects of medication.

What can be done about excessive gum growth when taking phenytoin (Dilantin)?

Excessive growth in gum tissue (gingival hyperplasia) often begins within two to three months after administration of phenytoin, for some individuals. The reason is not clear, and the phenomenon takes place only with phenytoin therapy. The condition reaches its most severe stages after about twelve to eighteen months of the therapy and is found far more often in children and adolescents than in adults. The tissue will return to normal size in approximately six months after phenytoin is stopped. Other side effects of phenytoin (for example, facial hair) are more lasting.

The condition is generally painless but can become unattractive. The gums can also become infected and irritated by calculus (tartar) or impacted food particles between the teeth and gums. Dilantin is probably inappropriate for adolescents undergoing orthodontic work, since the gum tissue covers the edge of the braces, giving rise to secondary infections. The condition may progress to the point where gingivectomy is required. In some cases, it is necessary to prescribe an alternative anticonvulsant.

Individuals with gum hyperplasia require a daily oral hygiene program involving frequent brushing, rinsing, and massage with a Water Pik or rubber tip. Dental floss is recommended. Professional dental care is recommended every three to four months, in the form of cleaning, scaling, and observation of the teeth and gums.

What should one do if the medication has been forgotten?

Anticonvulsant medication should be taken daily at convenient times as prescribed by the physician. It frequently happens that one is uncertain about whether the medication was given. In this case, it is generally advisable to give another dose as soon as the possible error is realized. Most persons will not have a seizure by missing one dose, but a frequent cause of increased seizure activity is reduced intake of medication. Though taking a second dosage may make the person temporarily drowsy, it is a better alternative than risking a seizure.

Most pharmacies carry medicine containers that hold a week's supply and are divided into seven compartments labeled Sunday, Monday, and so on. On Sunday the patient puts each day's supply of medicine into the appropriate compartment. At the end of each day that compartment should be empty if the person has remembered to take the medication. Many people find this an excellent way to keep track of the daily dose. If the medication has been forgotten during the day, it can simply be taken at bedtime.

What should we as parents do if we find we have run out of medication?

It frequently happens that parents suddenly find they are out of medication. This has often happened while traveling or on vacation and when not near the physician. In view of the danger to the child from missing his regular schedule, something must be done shortly. Seizures often become worse following a period when drugs are not given, and control is more difficult to reestablish. Also, the abrupt withdrawal of drugs can cause status epilepticus, which can be life-threatening.

Most pharmacists, even if off duty, are willing to refill a prescription in such an emergency. Emergency prescriptions for anticonvulsants may be obtained from any hospital emergency room by explaining the situation and providing the empty container so that the correct dosage may be continued. Pharmacists and physicians recognize the emergency and the dangers of a lack of medication in this situation and are usually willing to help.

My child stopped having seizures. Can I now stop giving the medication?

Sudden withdrawal of anticonvulsant medication involves a high risk of increasing seizure activity and status epilepticus. For some persons, the desire to stop the medication and the overconfidence caused by the absence of seizures lead to the temptation to discontinue the medication on their own. We have known of many such persons who wished to try to withdraw medication on their own, without consulting their physicians, in order to prove that they were no longer susceptible to seizures. This is especially true when one has been seizure-free for a relatively long period of time.

Remember that anticonvulsants do not cure epilepsy. They are designed to control the abnormal electrical discharges in the brain that result in seizures, and they usually do that job as long as they continue to be taken. If the epilepsy is under complete control for several years — usually three to five — the physician may attempt to remove the medication by gradually reducing the drug dosage, after a thorough discussion of the potential problems and with the patient's approval. This process of medication change should be done only under the close supervision of the physician.

What are the major factors to keep in mind about medication?

The following guidelines are important for home treatment with anticonvulsants:

1. Adhere faithfully to the prescribed medication schedule; that is, don't increase or decrease without consulting the physician.
2. Never discontinue the medication abruptly.
3. Obtain special instructions for times of stress or during illness.
4. Report any unusual symptoms, such as excessive sleepiness, difficulty in walking, change in behavior or seizure pattern, to the physician.
5. Do not allow young children to take their own medication without supervision.
6. Discuss any problems or side effects of the medication thoroughly with the physician either in person or by phone. If there are problems involved, it is better to talk about them and work with the physician to obtain the best control of the seizures with the fewest side effects from the medication.

7. Consider obtaining a container divided into compartments for the seven days of the week to make it easier to remember that the correct amount of medication has been taken.

Is it necessary to give the medication at the same time each day?

It is important to establish a routine for taking the medication, following the prescription as to the amount and number of times per day. The routine is normally set up around meals (either directly before or after), primarily so that taking the medication is more easily remembered. However, it is generally not necessary to give the medication at an *exact* time each day.

For many teenagers and adults, the entire dose of phenobarbital or phenytoin may be given at one time if so prescribed by the physician, to avoid the necessity of taking medication while at school or at work.

Why is it important to shake the bottle each time liquid medication is given?

On the surface, this question might seem rather trivial. However, in actual practice, shaking the bottle *does* make a difference in the dosage. As the liquid sits, the suspension will break down, leaving the filler at the top while the medication settles to the bottom of the bottle. Shaking redistributes the anticonvulsant medication evenly again. If the bottle is not shaken each time, the same number of spoonfuls given when the bottle is full, half-full, and near-empty will have surprisingly different amounts of medication. Therefore, you may actually be giving only a little medication or a heavy dose while still following the instructions on the bottle. This can cause the blood level of medication to drop when less medication is given and may result in seizure activity.

The only way to make certain each teaspoonful has the same measure of anticonvulsant medication is to shake the bottle vigorously each time.

Which is the more desirable form of medication for a child to take, liquid or tablets?

Most physicians prefer to prescribe tablets or capsules as soon as the child is able to swallow them with ease and safety. Tablets may even be crushed and given in baby food to the very young. Tablets and capsules provide a more accurate means of assuring that the child gets a correct dosage. Problems of liquid suspension were discussed in the previous question. Also, tablets can be carried more conveniently and are far less expensive than liquid medication.

Will prolonged use of anticonvulsant medication tend to make my child drug-addicted?

No. A number of follow-up studies have shown that children who took anticonvulsant drugs did not have addiction problems, either as children or in adulthood. Children who regularly take prescription anticonvulsants do not show any tendency to overmedication or to appear to want or to need other drugs. In fact, quite the reverse is true. In talking to many teenagers with epilepsy, our experience has been that the young people are looking forward to the day they can stop taking anticonvulsant medication and are far less interested than their peers in taking any other drugs.

Is medication for seizure control expensive?

The cost of anticonvulsant medication depends upon the type of drug, strength, and dosage. There is a wide range of prices, from as low as $2 per hundred pills to as high as $24. Some of the newer drugs such as Tegretol and Depakene are the most expensive.

From a survey conducted in 1974, the EFA found the average cost of anticonvulsants to be $178 per person per year. The same survey in 1977 showed the cost to be $213. The EFA estimates that annual anticonvulsant drug sales in the United States amount to more than $110,000,000. Medication continues to be a major expense for those with epilepsy.

I understand there is a low-cost drug program available for persons with epilepsy. Is this true, and if so, is the quality adequate?

There is such a program, available to all members of the Epilepsy Foundation of America and their immediate families. The parent (or person with epilepsy) merely sends the physician's prescription to the EFA Pharmacy Service, Second and Main Streets, Madrid, Iowa 50156. The telephone number is (515) 795–2450. Be sure your name and address are on the back of the prescription. The physician can also call the service to prescribe an anticonvulsant or to authorize a refill. The prescriptions are normally filled and returned by first-class mail or UPS the same day they are received. Allow two weeks for delivery. The EFA recommends that new medications be ordered well in advance to avoid the risk of running out at home. The EFA pharmacy bills the customer when the medication is sent.

The quality of the medication is assured. The pharmacy is well stocked with all of the anticonvulsants in present use. A price list is available and can be obtained by writing directly to the EFA Pharmacy Service at the above address.

6

FAMILY ADJUSTMENTS

Our child's seizures are now controlled. Will everything now be all right?

This book does not promise the future will be perfect. Some of the literature written to encourage parents implies that control of seizures through medication somehow solves all other problems. We have seen parents become discouraged and disappointed when this did not happen. The situation could have been at least partially avoided with a broader understanding of the medical, psychological, social, and educational problems so often associated with epilepsy.

From our experience, most children with seizure disorders *do* experience some problems of a psychological, educational, social, or medical nature during the course of their epilepsy. These difficulties can be eliminated or minimized when the parents become knowledgeable, can anticipate potential problems, and have prepared themselves to deal with the major traumatic situations. Such parents can seek proper advice and work with professionals to get this preparation.

We didn't understand everything the doctor told us. What should we do?

Physicians and the professionals who routinely deal with a certain specialty often tend to use terms and phrases that are common to them but not understood by others. For some reason, most of us are reluctant or embarrassed to ask questions we feel everyone else knows, and we somehow assume that someone else might ask the question. Furthermore, especially during diagnosis, the results may be given quickly, and the parents might not be in a condition to listen attentively.

Parents have a right as well as a duty to understand clearly everything they are being told, and it is their responsibility to ask repeatedly until they do fully understand, even if it requires a separate conference. No professional will be upset if parents ask for a point to be explained further, since the answer may be important to the child's future.

Are there some basic guidelines for raising a child with seizure disorders?

The principles or guidelines for raising one child are, in general, the same as for raising another. Children with seizure disorders are more like than unlike other children, and except in certain cases the universal principles of child-rearing are applicable to all. Each of the following general guidelines will be developed at greater length in questions covered later in this chapter.

1. *Treat the child normally.* Make only those exceptions that are absolutely necessary for safety. Allow the child to grow and take risks like other children, and to participate in activities with other children. Do not protect the child from other people or from situations.

2. *Be honest with yourself* about the seizure condition and your child's problems. Do not minimize the problems, but do not overreact to them, either. With a full acceptance of the situation, realistic expectations can be maintained.

3. *Build successful experiences* in your child's life. Make sure the child has an opportunity to do well in some area. Help the child develop his talents. Teach him how to deal with problems. The problems a child has learned to overcome are soon forgotten, while the problems a parent solves for the child remain with him always.

4. *Keep your child healthy.* This is a goal worth working for. Provide adequate nutrition, rest, and exercise. Do not dwell on the seizures by letting them be considered the most important aspect about your child. Rather than anxiously awaiting the next seizure, spend the same amount of time and concern building a healthy mind and body in your child.

5. *Explain the seizure condition to your child* when he is ready to understand the concept. Develop an open relationship with your child in a home atmosphere in which the child feels comfortable and secure. When this relationship is established, anything affecting you and the child can be discussed.

6. *Do not make an issue of the medication,* but maintain a matter-of-fact attitude about it, being sure that the daily routine is followed automatically.

7. *Maintain the family equilibrium.* Do not give or permit preferential treatment to the child with a seizure disorder. The other siblings, and even the spouse, often feel left out when one parent gives a disproportionate amount of time to one who is handicapped. Take planned breaks together, without the children, on occasional evenings or weekends. All parents need this respite occasionally to maintain the equilibrium that keeps a family balanced.

8. *Seek proper consultation and assistance when needed,* such as during periods of continued seizures, poor school performance, emotional problems, marital or family adjustment problems. Do not try to do everything alone. Rather, find the professionals who have experience and knowledge to help. Develop a friendship with a parent who has a child with a seizure disorder similar to that of your child, in order to share mutual concerns.

These principles and others are elaborated upon in this chapter. We consider the family relationships and adjustments to be the most vital aspect of the entire issue, perhaps second in importance only to the actual medical control of the seizures. The child and family who have developed and maintained a strong relationship can withstand any crisis. The family that can share a problem is perhaps the only family fully capable of sharing triumph.

Should a child's seizure condition be discussed in the presence of the other siblings?

We recommend that you do so. It has been our experience that the other children of the family are also anxious and concerned about the condition, and they most probably have less information about epilepsy than the parents. They know the child has been seen by doctors for diagnosis or treatment. If the results are not discussed openly in understandable language and their questions go unanswered, they will assume the worst and may not trust an accurate explanation later. A frank discussion will not upset the other children as much as silence or quick, superficial answers. A sibling may worry that *he* may also start having seizures. With concern and understanding, the siblings can help the child with seizures.

If the problems are not discussed in the family, you should examine whether the reason is your rejection or guilt, rather than protection of the children. Family communication is important at all times. The test of the solidarity of the family comes during such a crisis. Apprehension, tension, and fear are normal for parents during the period of diagnosis and early treatment. If the other children are aware of your reactions, they, too, will soon realize that it is all right for them to have and to express these emotions.

Will punishing my child induce a seizure?

You must make every effort not to treat a child differently because he has had seizures. Remember that the attitude of the child will generally reflect your attitude. Parental oversolicitude, hostility, rejection, or even worse, pity, may occur in any family, but if they do, they need to be remedied and changed. Either to punish or to pamper a child because he has seizures tends only to produce a child who has more seizures *and* a behavior disorder. The behavior disorder often becomes more of a problem than the seizures.

Occasionally, a seizure may happen after you have disciplined your child. This may make you as a parent feel uncomfortable, but it is insufficient justification to change your general disciplinary procedures. If an infraction warrants discipline for the other children, it also does for the child with a seizure disorder. Children in a family must be treated in the same manner. Otherwise, the child with the seizure disorder soon discovers he is "different," and can learn to manipulate parents and siblings.

If a child gains undue attention due to seizures, he may soon learn to "fake" such seizures, or, in some cases, even bring on a legitimate seizure in an effort to gain his own way. The sooner a child learns that he is treated no differently from his siblings, the happier and better adjusted all in the family become.

Is it necessary to keep a record of the seizures?

A record may be required for a brief time by the physician in order to evaluate the effect of a drug or to examine the specific environmental influences on a seizure disorder. It is important that the physician know the approximate number of seizures, but the exact frequency and time are rarely required.

Extended and detailed records are generally not necessary and may even set up attitudes that may be harmful for the person with seizures. Records of this type only serve to keep the seizures in the awareness of the whole family. The family should be cautioned not to watch for seizures or to inquire whether the person had a seizure, but to stress normal activity and engage in family life without undue emphasis on the seizures.

I was advised not to overprotect my child, yet he needs special care. Isn't it better to "overprotect" than to risk an accident?

Ever since David Levy wrote his classic *Maternal Overprotection* in 1943, parents have gradually become aware of the dangers in doing too much for a child. This of course applies to fathers as well as mothers, and the disastrous importance of the dangers of overprotection cannot be overemphasized.

Almost instinctively, most parents tend to protect their young. When a child is handicapped, there is an even greater tendency to go out of our way to ensure the child's safety, all too often at the expense of the child's feelings of independence. Many parents pamper a child because of mixed emotions that the child should have everything possible to compensate for his condition. They often fear that an emotional upset could precipitate a seizure, not realizing that failure to set guidelines often leads to feelings of inferiority and resentment in the child.

For some reason, our culture continues to rob its children of the opportunity to develop true responsibility by making decisions for them. This is true of parents of most children; we seem to prefer to tell them things they could better find out for themselves. The overprotected child suffers from perhaps the greatest of handicaps —loss of independence and initiative.

Of course we need to remind the young child of certain acts that are necessary for his health and safety, such as taking medication regularly. The utmost care, however, must be taken to make the handicapped child independent as soon as possible, and to see that he is treated as any other child.

Should I restrict my child's physical activities?

Yes — if necessary, though the way it is done is of prime importance. Constant restrictions leave the child with feelings of being "different" from other children, one of the things we try to avoid. It is better to encourage positive actions and interests in the child. Let him know you are proud of his accomplishments and guide him into endeavors in which he has a good chance for success. With the young child, especially, make sure you are proud of his efforts. The general guide should be to emphasize what the child can do rather than what should not be done because of the disorder.

Generally, physical activity favorably affects the person with a seizure disorder. The person with epilepsy is usually encouraged to participate in most of the physical activities enjoyed by others. Parents need to allow their children to play and exercise in a normal manner. In fact, people experience fewer seizures during activity than during rest. Many have their seizures only during sleep, and often EEG abnormalities can be detected only during a drowsy state.

Obviously, the person with uncontrolled seizures should not perform activities that would be dangerous in the event of a fall (mountain climbing, motorcycle riding, high diving, hang gliding, and so on). Most authorities advise swimming only under supervision. Otherwise, activities that are appropriate for the child's age should be encouraged.

Since all activities have some risk of injury to all children or adults — whether they have epilepsy or not — any restriction should be made only on the basis of avoiding those situations which would produce serious injury.

Many parents assume that they should not allow an adolescent to participate in body contact sports such as soccer, football, or boxing at school, for fear that an injury to the head would increase the possibility of seizures. There is no clear evidence that a head injury of the type that might result from body contact would aggravate a seizure disorder. These sports are possible with medical clearance.

Is swimming advisable for a child with seizures?

This is a difficult decision, since swimming is healthful, pleasurable, and considered a normal activity for children, and normalcy is one of our chief goals. Yet, seizures do pose a major hazard should they occur in the water. The topic should be discussed with a physician, the parents, and the child or adolescent with epilepsy.

Strict rules prohibiting swimming are necessary if seizures are uncontrolled. If the seizures are under control, swimming is possible with certain precautions. No person with epilepsy should swim alone; he should swim with a buddy under supervision of an adult or lifeguard and avoid physical exhaustion. Children in the water, near a pool, or in a boat should wear life jackets. Young children prone to seizures should not be left alone in the bathtub.

The adults should organize the swimming event so that the child can have fun, but they must see that the safety rules are obeyed.

What can be done if the child is subject to ridicule?

Other children may be cruel to a child with a convulsive disorder, and as parents you will want to prepare your child for this possibility. Most children can understand a simple explanation of epilepsy and can be made to realize that many people simply have not had the chance to learn about seizures. You may want to arm your child with certain verbal comebacks when he is dealing in a friendly way with the tormentors.

Your child should be made to know that the statements of other children are usually made for effect, and that if he does not respond in the expected manner, the effect is lost and the unwanted comments tend not to be repeated. Also, if your child has developed friendships and gained acceptance by a peer group, any ridicule or thoughtless remarks by them will have fewer disturbing consequences.

It is usually helpful for the parent or teacher to talk with the offenders, quietly and confidentially. A special kit for teachers as well as parents (Epilepsy School Alert program) is available for just such purposes and is described in the section of this book related to education.

What are the pitfalls of lack of parental acceptance of the condition?

There are a number of parental reactions to epilepsy that can have devastating effects for the child. There is a common tendency for parents to overprotect their children (discussed more fully in a previous question), and this protective love too often results in the child's getting a disproportionate amount of attention, toys, special foods, and the like. Often, the child with epilepsy is allowed to do as he pleases, for fear a denial may bring on a seizure. We know of many children with seizures who have been spoiled by such an attitude. In some cases, the child may be regarded as sick and in need of protection from ordinary play, or forced to rest, conserve his energy, or require inordinate protection from germs or sources of infection. The child is often not allowed to play with other children or to engage in social activities, resulting in a lack of ability to deal with people. In other cases, a parent may reject the child with epilepsy.

All of these parental attitudes or situations carry the serious risk of developing behavior disorders or neuroses in the child, which can be far more debilitating and much more difficult to control than the seizures themselves.

If any of these pitfalls describe the reactions of members of your family, seek assistance in correcting the situation as soon as possible. Seek a counselor with knowledge of convulsive disorders and experience in working with families.

What should we tell other people about epilepsy?

Everyone, especially parents, should know some basic facts about epilepsy. If the general public, primarily employers, had increased knowledge of the disorder, much of the misinformation and prejudice would diminish and living with seizures would be made much easier. What you tell others about your child's condition may well be their only information; thus, providing even the basics may be most helpful.

In general, everyone should be aware of the following facts about epilepsy:

1. Epilepsy is not an infectious disease. It is a symptom of a disorder of the brain, and therefore it cannot be transmitted by contact with someone who has it.
2. Epilepsy is a common neurological problem shared by more than two million Americans.
3. Epilepsy can affect anyone at any age. It does not mean that the person is mentally retarded or mentally ill.
4. Epilepsy has many forms, from severe convulsions to momentary lapses of attention.
5. Epilepsy can be treated, and most persons can lead normal lives.
6. The psychological problems, social prejudice, and employment barriers that so often accompany epilepsy are usually far more handicapping than the seizures themselves.

It is unrealistic to expect the people you come in contact with to be fully knowledgeable and understanding of the disorder, and most people (though they might not admit it) do not know even the six basic facts listed above. You can help raise the level of understanding by direct communication, by giving or leaving literature for people to read, or by working with the local epilepsy society in public education projects. Do not overestimate the knowledge most people have about epilepsy. Most know very little and need to have their knowledge gap corrected!

I have heard that our attitude as parents is one of the most important factors in our child's "normalization." Is this right?

As we mentioned, children are greatly influenced by the attitudes and reactions of their parents and other significant adults. It is generally recognized that early life experiences and relationships with the family are of prime importance, since they assist in the development of personality, attitudes, and formation of self-worth. Since most seizure disorders originate in early childhood, the parental reaction is a primary determinant of the child's reaction to the disorder and to himself.

The most important thing parents can do is to direct their efforts toward raising a normal child within the limits of the disability. This requires a matter-of-fact attitude toward the seizures, love, a relaxed and supportive atmosphere, and the normal social and physical activities enjoyed by the other children.

An essential element in providing a natural family atmosphere is the acceptance of the seizure disorder by all the family members. Families who live in constant dread of "another seizure" will quickly communicate this fear to the child. Parents who have examined their own reactions to the seizure disorder and have achieved a general state of acceptance are in the best position to pay full attention to maintaining a family environment that is supportive and rewarding to their child.

I admit that I still worry about what other people think.
Exactly how does the general public feel about epilepsy?

This question has been answered every five years in the Gallup polls, with a surprising and reassuring change in the public attitude revealed each time the poll has been taken. In 1949, for example, when the attitudes on epilepsy were first queried, nearly one fourth of the people polled stated that they would not wish their child to attend school or play with a child who might have seizures. By 1974, the number had shrunk to one in twenty. Though this percentage is still too high, it does show a great change.

In 1949, 13 percent of the people considered epilepsy as a form of insanity, compared with 2 percent in 1974. In 1949, less than half the people polled felt those with epilepsy should be regularly employed; in 1974, more than four out of five people favored regular employment.

Granted, these statistics still show a dearth of general information about epilepsy on the part of the general public. However, considering the dramatic change in the past twenty-five years and the Nationwide Plan for Action (see the Epilogue), we should expect growth in understanding to continue, and at an even faster rate.

What is self-esteem?

Self-esteem refers to how a person feels about himself—his own attitudes and self-judgment about his worth (or lack of worth) as a person. A person with high esteem might make statements such as "I'm glad I'm me," "I can do things," "People like me," or "I am loved even when I'm bad." These statements reflect the general attitude that the child or adult feels comfortable about himself. This is the essence of a desirable self-picture. The attitude is not one of vanity or conceit, but one of genuine confidence and positive identity.

Authorities (such as Arthur Combs) feel that we are virtually compelled to behave in keeping with our self-concept or self-esteem. We simply tend to behave as *we* see ourselves. Self-esteem is also heavily influenced by how we believe *others* see us. Though all children must have positive feelings of self-worth, this attitude is of even greater importance to the handicapped child, who may already have developed a low self-concept.

How can we as parents develop self-confidence and positive self-esteem in our child?

Children develop a self-concept in their early years that tends to evolve and be maintained throughout their lives. The child's respect for himself as a person will be carried with him everywhere and will influence practically everything he does in life. Assisting your child to develop positive self-esteem is one of the most important functions you can have as a parent.

The parents are the major factor in the development of the self-image in their children. These parental reflections become some of the first and most powerful impressions the child ever experiences. It is generally held that by age five, the child's basic self-concept is developed, and the child has a relatively fixed opinion about himself as a person. This opinion is learned from the degree to which the child feels valued by persons of significance to him, primarily the parents, but also baby-sitters, preschool teachers, or grandparents. The child simply learns to value himself to the same extent that he feels valued by persons he regards as important.

The child with high self-esteem will be able to cope better with peers when he enters school and will also be better able to cope with problems that occur in connection with seizures. The child automatically modifies his feelings by his early experiences at home and in school, which tend to affect his school performance significantly. In adolescence, one's peers replace parents and teachers as the significant persons who modify feelings of self-worth. In this respect, an adequate self-concept and feelings of peer approval are even more vital to the adolescent with seizure disorders.

There are some specific steps in assisting your child's development of self-esteem:

1. Set aside a short time each day *just* for listening to your child. It need be only ten or fifteen minutes, as long as it is devoted entirely to listening to your child without inter-

rupting, or letting your mind wander, or doing it as a "duty," or worrying about something else. This time should not be just when the child misbehaves, but it should be a "special time" established purely because the child is an important person.

2. Express pleasure and pride in your child. Be encouraging and do not belittle the child's foolish aspirations or ambitions. A psychologist of our acquaintance tells the interesting anecdote of having heard every day from his mother what a joy he was to her, and how she wished she had a dozen more just like him. He said that he was in his twenties before he realized that he had been the last of seven boys being raised during the heart of the Depression by his widowed mother, and that surely a dozen more "just like him" would have been almost an impossibility. However, he remembered all through his youth that he had considered himself just what his mother had "needed."

3. Give your child experiences of success and personal achievement. Be careful not to expect more than the child can actually perform. Give recognition for accomplishments before family and friends. It can be very gratifying for a child to hear his parents proudly sharing his accomplishments with friends. The child with a good self-concept can easily learn to accept failure when he knows that regardless of his performance in a certain skill, he is accepted as a person.

4. Relax when you are with your child. A parent filled with tension reflects that tension, and the young child somehow assumes the tension concerns him, rather than a particular problem the parent may have. Furthermore, parental concerns and fears about seizures will be transmitted nonverbally, even when not mentioned, to the child.

What should I do if my child lies or steals?

Most children lie or steal at some time during their childhood, and there is no evidence that seizures have anything to do with this natural phenomenon. When it happens, remain calm and look for the cause rather than the punishment. A child may steal to acquire a desired object or to feel loved. The child may steal to buy or give things to another child in an attempt to buy friendship or status. In a sense, and perhaps at a more sophisticated level, many parents do the same. A child may lie to cover a misdeed, may fabricate experiences to gain status by impressing friends, or may subconsciously see the lie as a means of bolstering the ego. Deal with the child fairly and without emotion. Explain the consequences of the lie or theft. The child can simply return whatever was stolen without unnecessary feelings of shame or guilt, or can repay the loss from his allowance, not as punishment per se, but as a natural consequence of the act. The best way to prevent a recurrence is to make sure the child understands what was wrong, and that the child does not lose his positive feelings of worth as an individual.

As mentioned, every child at one time or another will lie or steal. Whether this becomes an isolated event or a behavior pattern to be continued depends largely on how the parents handle the situation. By no means should the child be branded as thief or liar, especially in front of others. The more insecure the child, the greater the tendency to repeat the very acts he thought brought him recognition.

Should our child have chores?

Absolutely! Every child, regardless of ability level or handicap, should have chores appropriate to his abilities. The chores should involve a regular set of tasks, performance of which is expected without reminders from you. Start with the self-help tasks, such as picking up clothes and making the bed, and gradually add family tasks (like feeding the pets or taking out the garbage) as the child matures. You might even give an added incentive or reward, whether it be in the form of a compliment or something more tangible, when the chores are done without reminders. What you are striving for here is independence on the part of the child, and the goal is self-initiated behavior.

Do not allow members of the family to make special allowances or excuses for the child with seizures, or to permit him to get out of responsibilities that he is capable of performing. Routine performance of chores is a vital part of the development of responsibility, without which no child can have an adequate self-concept.

What can I do to help develop my child's speech?

There are a number of ways in which a parent can aid a child's speech development at home. First, and perhaps most important, be a good listener when the child speaks. The fact that a child is communicating is far more important than the *way* he talks, and a child's speech tends to be less inhibited when he knows he is listened to. Never try to correct the child's speech when he is talking. We have known of parents who would actually interrupt the child in the middle of a sentence with statements such as "You are talking too fast; try it again more slowly," or "I just can't hear you when you mumble your words." The child who is made to feel self-conscious about his speech tends to develop more poor speech habits than the child who knows he has a ready and interested audience.

Encourage the child to use complete sentences as much as possible, rather than answering with a single word. Do not allow the child to point when asking for something if he knows the word. Use adult conversation and discourage baby talk. Never use baby talk yourself. This all too common practice merely prolongs poor speech habits in children, though many parents feel it is cute and "accepting." Slowly repeat words you want the child to understand. Correct mistakes by merely answering with the correct word, without commenting on the child's mistake.

Speech games can be fun for the child, and can improve his oral expression at the same time. To be effective, these must literally be games and not seen by the child as speech lessons. The child must be absorbed in the game rather than in his speech. The games listed below can be adapted according to the child's ability (best for ages three to ten):

Rhymes. Take turns finding words that rhyme with a starter word, such as *sat* — cat, mat, fat, bat, etc.

Riddles. Make up riddles with the names of animals, foods, jobs, etc.:

I hammer nails and saw boards. I am a —.
I have four legs and fur, and I purr. I am a —.
I am cold, I taste good, and am eaten from a cone. I am —.

Twenty Questions. The child must guess the identity of a person, place, or thing by asking twenty questions or less, which must be answered by the adult with only a "yes" or a "no."

What happened game. Begin with a situation and have the child make up an ending. "I went to the circus and got lost. What do you think happened? What do you think I saw?"

You can help build a child's vocabulary by encouraging him to read, by letting him watch television, and by talking about experiences, even while riding in the car. A child learns new words more easily when he has seen or had an experience associated with the word or concept. The child who has been out with his parents picks up new words and develops better speech than the child who remains at home watching television alone or without conversation. The child who has grown up with word games invariably develops better speech and language patterns than the child who has not had these experiences. We have known of parents who helped develop their child's vocabulary and speech through the simple technique of cutting pictures out of magazines, pasting them on plain cards, and talking about the pictures. Older children or adults with difficulty in speech need comprehensive speech and language examinations.

For further information we recommend the book *Teach Your Child to Talk,* described in Appendix B, as an excellent resource.

When and how much should my child be told of his condition?

The child should be told of his condition as soon as he is able to recognize that something is wrong and can understand a simple explanation. The description should be accurate and appropriate to the child's age and mental development. A lengthy and detailed description of epilepsy is not necessary and may needlessly frighten the child.

Generally, a four-year-old is capable of understanding that he has "fainting spells" or "convulsions," which will require follow-up treatment. The child can then understand why he must continue to go to the doctor and have repeated blood samples. Older children can use the term "epilepsy" and "seizures." The child should know that these terms are interchangeable even if they are not all used in the household, because he may hear them from other sources. As the child reaches puberty (and often before), he can be given greater details about the disorder and the conditions that can either assist or aggravate his own situation.

The explanation of the condition is considered best when it comes from the parents, but it may be supplemented by the physician or other helping professionals known to the child. A parent who is severely upset by the condition is usually in a poor position to communicate these facts to the child, and, conversely, the accepting parent is the best one to give the explanation. If the parents are relatively comfortable with the condition, the child will be also.

A brief explanation is preferable to no knowledge, since many young children who were not told for "their own protection" have developed emotional problems from assuming they had some unknown disease that physicians were unable to discover, or may fear they have a terminal illness that the parents do not wish to discuss. It is better for the child to know the disorder has been diagnosed and that the doctor is trying to find the right medicine for him.

We suggest that children who are explaining or discussing their disorder with friends use terms such as "black out" or "pass out." These terms are generally understood and accepted without negative feelings.

Are my other children apt to be adversely affected by any special treatment of our child with epilepsy?

One could almost categorically state that the brothers or sisters of a child who is handicapped are *never* affected by the mere presence of a handicapped child's condition, by itself. They *do* react, however, to the attitudes of the parents toward the handicapped child. If the siblings suspect that the child with epilepsy is receiving special treatment they do not receive, or that he is given certain liberties they are not, or that the parents are overly concerned or solicitous, the children are quick to pick this up and to find means of receiving the same treatment. It is not uncommon, especially for very young children, to emulate the behavior of their handicapped sibling in an effort to gain the special attention they feel the sibling is receiving. We have even known of children who simulated a seizure in order to gain the attention received by their brother or sister with epilepsy.

It has been a major premise of this book that children with epilepsy are far more *like* than unlike the other children, and that they must receive as nearly identical treatment as possible. This is not only for the benefit of children with seizures, but for the siblings and parents as well. Children, handicapped or not, will readily needle a parent at any time if such behavior will gain attention.

How can we avoid jealousy between our child with epilepsy and our other children?

Each child in a family is important and deserves an equal share of the attention, discipline, responsibility, and love. The presence of some jealousy is common among children. However, jealousy brought about by excessive attention to the child with seizures can result in discord within the entire family. Siblings deprived of attention from the parents, or of activities they cannot attend because of the handicapped child, will become resentful of the child with epilepsy.

There are some general guidelines for handling and preventing jealousy or sibling rivalry:

1. Avoid comparisons of one child with another.
2. Make sure you *are* being fair to all the children. Families often tend to give a disproportionate amount of time to the one who needs special help. Remember that all the children need help and deserve a share of support and attention.
3. Have a private time for each child in the family. Even a parent with many children can spend five minutes alone with each child every day.
4. Require all children to perform household chores. Do not make an exception for the child with epilepsy, but give each child appropriate tasks, dependent upon his or her abilities.

5. Never be afraid to tell each child daily that he is loved. True, children know when and whether they are loved, but they also need to be told. No child is too old to hear this message.

The child with epilepsy should be given no more favors than the others, nor should he be left out of family activities because of the condition. Every child needs a secure place in the family. Sometimes jealousy on the part of the children is a clue that the parents or relatives are giving the handicapped child more attention than is good for all concerned.

Should we take our child out socially with us, even though we realize that he might have a seizure?

Absolutely, provided the outing is not one that might prove dangerous to the child. The fact that a child is subject to seizures has nothing to do with his need to accompany his parents to the same places where his brothers or sisters are free to go. We have known of parents whose true motive in not taking their child with them socially was the fear of embarrassment to themselves or their friends, rather than actual concern for the child. The rule of thumb should be to take your child wherever you would take your other children, provided there is no physical danger to the child.

Should I send my child to camp?

Yes. Parents have no need to be afraid to send a child or young adult with epilepsy to a special camp with trained staff. (Directories of special camps are listed in Appendix A.) Also information on local camps capable of handling persons with seizure disorders may be available from the school, or local parents' group.

Many parents find the thought of separation from their child very difficult and are unduly concerned that the child might have a seizure. The special camps have a staff accustomed to dealing with seizures — in fact, that is the reason for special camps. Normally, a child is eligible to attend camp if the seizures are reasonably under control. The child does not need to be seizure-free. The parent is usually requested to inform the camp personnel of the normal frequency of seizures, the dosage of medication, and the physician to contact in case of emergency. The parent, of course, sends the needed medication along with the child, with adequate dosage for the camp period.

Camp can (and should) be an adventure and a growth experience for the child. We have seen dramatic changes as a result of the companionship, excitement, and independence fostered by even one week of special camp. The child's attendance at camp also provides a needed respite for the parents and other members of the family.

Does bed-wetting accompany a seizure disorder?

Bed-wetting or enuresis is the involuntary passage of urine by a child over three years of age. The cause is usually emotional and is sustained by habit. Enuresis can occur in children with epilepsy as well as in other children. Occasionally, enuresis is due to an infection of the bladder or urinary tract, and it is well to check this first before considering other possible causes.

In some cases, the enuresis may be the result of incontinence from a seizure at night that went unnoticed. The treatment is dependent upon the cause and should be done in consultation with the physician and psychologist.

I cannot help pitying my child when he has seizures. Is this wrong?

One of the greatest injustices we can do to any person is to pity him. This is especially true of the handicapped child, who needs, above all, to be treated as a normal child. Pity is basically a selfish emotion — one in which we are actually pitying ourselves. The one who pities a child inevitably tries to protect him from responsibility, decisions, and the like, thereby perpetuating the child's inabilities. All children become overly dependent if the parent permits himself this indulgent emotion. We must remember that a handicap is not as disabling as the reactions toward it by those around the child. Attitudes of pity cause a child to see himself as unfortunate.

How can I relax when I know my child could have a seizure?

A common problem for parents of a child with epilepsy is that they live in dread of the next seizure. Though the concern is shared by both parents, the mother is more often the one who provides much of the home care and is more apt to be present when the seizure does occur.

Actually, there is little you as a parent *can* do to prevent a seizure once the child is under proper treatment. Worry becomes cyclic, and, rather than helping anyone, worry affects not only the child but the entire family as well. Recognizing that the care and concern of a child with epilepsy can be demanding and sometimes draining, we suggest the following techniques.

Take time for yourself, and do some of the things you have wanted to do. Remember that your physical and mental health are important to the overall well-being of the family. We know of one parent with very modest means who nevertheless took an afternoon a week away from the home and the child, having made arrangements with a neighbor to be present. Sometimes the mother did little but walk around the city park, but it was *her* time, to do with as she wished. Whether it is playing bridge, tennis, reading, or merely taking a bath, you need a regular time that is your own.

Seek training in self-relaxing techniques, if needed, from a psychologist or other qualified professional. You will find that once you learn the basic techniques, you will be able to use them whenever you wish.

Remember, if your goal is to help your child, the best way to do this is to help yourself by providing a calm and relaxed home atmosphere. Stress may bring on seizures — relaxation often inhibits them. Older adolescents and adults with seizures who are chronically tense can also benefit from self-relaxation training, once they realize that everything that should be done to control the seizures *has* been done.

The Scriptures seem to imply that one with seizures may be "possessed." Is it possible that God could be punishing us for past sins by seizures in our child?

Almost none of today's theologians would hold this position. In the past, however, persons with seizures were often regarded as "possessed." Because the causes and treatment of epilepsy were unknown, family members often felt that God was punishing them. It seemed easy to attach a moral or theological significance to that which they could not understand, especially when certain scriptures could be interpreted as referring to a condition similar to epilepsy (see, for instance, Matthew 8:28–33, in which Jesus cast out the "demons" from two men). In fact, a recent Gallup poll showed that 4 percent of the population still consider epilepsy as some sort of a curse.

With the advances in medical knowledge as to the causes and treatment of epilepsy, one should not consider seizures as punishment any more than any other disorder.

What if the husband and wife should disagree on what is best for the child?

Whenever the parents disagree, the child will become aware of the discord. Parents will naturally disagree on occasion, but not, we hope, in the presence of the child. Parents need to take the time to talk through the difficulties as soon as they are apparent and to agree on a mutual plan. If great disparity in opinion persists, seek guidance from a counselor or physician regarding the issue.

Sometimes a parent will make a personal commitment for the care and protection of the child with seizures, to the exclusion of the other family members and in opposition to the spouse. This is a troublesome situation for the child as well as for the marriage. The spouse will often resent such actions. When this is the case, professional help is needed, since a unilateral focus on the child's needs puts a major strain on the marriage.

In general, what would the parents of children with epilepsy like the public to know?

There have been a number of surveys of parental attitudes in both Canada and the United States, which suggest that the primary concern of the parents of children with epilepsy is the lack of knowledge and concern of the general public. A recent Canadian study found a great many parents unwilling to discuss openly the problems their children had encountered. The author of this study found that many of the parents gave no reason for their reluctance to participate in the study, and the writer assumed it was due to the stigma attached to the disorder.

A subsequent study found the primary concern of the parents was the need for public information and education. They wanted to bring epilepsy more "into the light." In connection with this need for public awareness, a 1974 Gallup poll found a surprisingly large number (approximately five million people) who still believed epilepsy to be caused by such bizarre factors as demonic possession, radioactive fall-out, or exotic foods and beverages.

Does the person with epilepsy normally have fears in connection with the disorder?

The person with epilepsy may experience a variety of emotional reactions with regard to the recurrence of seizures. The reactions may range from mere annoyance to severe personality disturbances. Much depends on the person's attitude and knowledge about the disorder and the attitude of others.

The most common emotional reactions to the disorder are anxiety, depression, and fear. Uncontrolled or partially controlled seizures can leave the person discouraged or depressed about the "unfairness" of the condition. Fear of the loss of consciousness and lack of control is a particularly disturbing problem that tends to leave many persons tense and generally apprehensive ("free-floating anxiety"). Unfortunately, any prolonged state of anxiety may have the effect of lowering the threshold for a seizure, thus tending to make the situation even worse.

A further complicating factor is the concern about the public awareness of epilepsy. Many persons with seizure disorders are aware of negative attitudes some people have regarding seizures and are easily embarrassed about identifying their condition. Many, because of this, have attempted to conceal their condition from friends or associates. Such persons are then forced to live in an increased state of tension from fear of being "exposed" by an attack. Such increased tension naturally increases the possibility of an attack; thus, it is far wiser not to attempt to hide the condition.

We have known of parents who attempted to keep the condition a secret by keeping their child at home most of the time. This physical and emotional isolation may lead to far more lasting emotional problems than any momentary embarrassment a seizure might have produced. Isolation or secrecy also prevents the opportunity to encourage positive public attitudes.

Should we belong to a local epilepsy society?

There are a number of good reasons for joining a chapter of a local epilepsy society. First, the group is composed of people with similar concerns — family members, persons with epilepsy, business and professional persons interested in the field — all working for improved conditions at the local level. Many such groups sponsor local projects.

Second, the meetings often have a speaker or discuss new information or literature in the field, and you are assured of being kept up to date regarding the latest in research or techniques concerning the care of your child. Special pamphlets or books may be available at the meeting or shared by members.

Third, you will meet people with similar problems. It is remarkable what therapy is provided by meeting other parents with difficulties you may have considered unique to you.

Fourth, the meetings will provide an opportunity to learn what is happening in the area of legislation. It is significant that *most* of the facilities for special children were developed purely as a result of parents' groups. Most professional educators are well aware of the influence of parents' groups on legislation that first was permissive, then became mandatory. The local chapter has a much stronger effect on legislators than an individual member does. You will find that legislators may be willing to come to a group meeting to listen to the concerns of the group, but may be reluctant to hear a single individual. Furthermore, much of the support for research and diagnostic centers is the direct result of organized and articulate groups concerned with epilepsy.

Even if you are not a "joiner," it would be well to go to several meetings so that you understand what the group is attempting to do. By all means, get your name on the mailing list.

Could we get practical help at a parents' group?

We have found that parents of children recently diagnosed as having a seizure disorder nearly always benefit in a practical way from group membership and attendance. The parents' group may be run by the special education department of the school system or the local epilepsy society chapter. Membership provides an opportunity to talk to other parents of handicapped children.

Often, parents feel they need to seek out a family with the exact problem they are facing, and have more confidence when receiving help from one in a similar situation. Actually, it is really not necessary to talk with someone with the *exact* problem, as one can benefit equally from hearing the experiences of those who have children with various handicaps. Parents are often surprised at how many similarities exist in a group with diversified disabilities. Though the disability may vary, the feelings and process of coping are often the same. Such groups offer the opportunity for support and advice, as well as the chance merely to talk to others about child-rearing. Many parents who feel they might have little to contribute do so more than they realize by sharing experiences at a group meeting.

How can I locate a parents' group?

There are currently more than 160 active chapters of the Epilepsy Foundation of America throughout the country, with more than 50,000 members. In addition to these chapters, there are countless splinter groups located in virtually every city in the United States and in other countries. For information about the nearest parents' group, you may contact the EFA headquarters (see Appendix A).

Other sources of information about parents' groups may be obtained through the local school district, family physician, or health department.

What about self-help groups?

Recently small groups of persons with epilepsy have started to meet together to exchange experiences and offer emotional support to one another through group discussion and personal caring. This can be an effective aid to someone having difficulty accepting the condition. These groups really focus on the everyday problems of coping with a seizure disorder.

For information on where to join such a group or how to organize one, contact Self-Help Center, 2040 Sheridan Road, Evanston, Illinois 60201, or your local epilepsy association.

Are there any organizations available for young adults with epilepsy?

A newly formed organization, the Epilepsy Youth Association, provides a way for teenagers and young adults to raise money and to have fun with dance marathons, walks, and a variety of activities. The Epilepsy Youth Association is a part of the Epilepsy Foundation of America.

EYA chapters are currently forming in many states; their programs include fund-raising, community service projects, public education, and counseling other young people. If no chapter exists in your area, contact the EFA for information on how to get one started. The EFA is eager to help and can provide information on the mechanics involved.

Are there books on epilepsy that my child could read?

Yes, and we have found this to be an excellent way for a child to gain a general understanding of just what is happening to him. You might read with the child and discuss the material later. Though individual reading by the child is not a substitute for an explanation by the parent or doctor, it can be valuable for answering questions the child had not thought to ask.

From our experience and communication with other professionals regarding interpreting epilepsy to children, we suggest the following material:

	Ages
Benjamin (comic book and film)	6 to 10
Because You Are My Friend (pamphlet and slide presentation)	7 to 12
What Everyone Should Know About Epilepsy (pamphlet)	7 to 12
Epilepsy, by Alvin and Virginia Silverstein	13 and older
Epilepsy, by Allen H. Middleton, Arthur A. Attwell, and Gregory O. Walsh	16 and older

The first four books and pamphlets are referred to in Appendixes B and C. Several films are also useful in interpreting to children and are listed in Appendix D, though of course it may be inconvenient to show a film to one child at a time. The slide presentation *Because You Are My Friend* is a notable exception and is well worth showing to a single child.

We have also listed various books of fiction in Appendix B. These stories about people with epilepsy present mild seizure disorders in a sensitive and understanding way and are considered to be excellent sources for adolescents who need this material.

Will my child be able to get married and have children?

The concern of every parent is a normal life for his child, and the answer to this question needs more than a superficial "yes, of course." Most children with epilepsy *can* be expected to lead a full life, including marriage and children if they desire. However, a few problems should be considered:

1. If mental retardation is present in addition to the seizure disorder, marriage and children may not be possible, depending upon the extent of the retardation.
2. If the child has experienced seizures that could not be controlled and are expected to continue, he or she might be less able to provide and care for a family.
3. A rare situation sometimes occurs in which pregnancy increases seizure activity for a woman with epilepsy, even to the point of a risk to her life. Most physicians generally advise against further pregnancies when such has proved to be the case.
4. The risk of passing on the disorder is greatest when there is a family history of epilepsy in both partners, especially if the seizures are of an idiopathic type that started early in life.

When one or both of the partners has a history of epilepsy, it is advisable to seek genetic counseling to assess the risks in having children. The ultimate decision, of course, rests with the couple.

The psychologist talked with us about the "stages" of growth in acceptance of the reality of seizure disorder in a child. What are the stages, and what can be done to promote adjustment?

From our experience, parents may go through several stages of adjustment to a child with a seizure disorder, often without realizing at the time the reactions they are experiencing. There is some variation, depending on whether the seizures develop in early childhood or later, and whether they are obvious to other people. Incidentally, these stages or phases of parental adjustment are common in most other disorders, as well as epilepsy. Few loving parents are so objective as to merely take their child's handicap as a matter of fact. It is not only normal but healthy as well for the parents to adjust gradually to a new and surprising condition in their child. The following is a brief outline of the common stages in the normal parental adjustment process to having a handicapped child.

Stage I: Shock and Confusion. The initial awareness that something is wrong with the child produces a specific kind of shock and anxiety. The reaction is accompanied by a feeling of helplessness. If the diagnosis is not made quickly, and knowledge about seizures given, the parents easily begin to worry and to become confused by fears. Nothing incapacitates people like fear. Parents in this condition cannot really listen to what they are told.

Stage II: Denial. Some parents refuse to accept the diagnosis and may seek another doctor. They will make statements such as, "That doctor saw my child for only five minutes, how can he be so sure?" "The tests must have been misinterpreted." "My child isn't retarded; that doctor is not an expert." Indeed this was the very pattern followed by one of the authors of this book when, several years ago, he searched for a doctor who would give him a favorable diagnosis about his own child. Frequently, a family will begin a frantic search for another doctor or another clinic to give a different answer or provide a "cure." Many parents are unable to accept the report that no cause can be identified for their child's seizures and lose confidence in doctors when told there is no cure, only control of the condition.

Stage III: Mourning. This stage is often present in parents who have an infant with seizures or a child who is mentally retarded. Not all parents experience this stage. It is here that the parents mourn the loss of the normalcy they expected in their child. All parents expect a normal, healthy baby without any handicap and are not prepared for seizures that they do not as yet understand. Parents who have difficulty progressing through this stage often feel self-pity and are not fully able to help their child. The birth of any handicapped child damages the self-esteem and confidence of the parents.

Stage IV: Anger and Guilt. Anger is a frequent emotion often directed toward the doctor who made the diagnosis, one's spouse, or oneself and emerges when the denial stage is over. A parent may be angry at God, feeling that he or she has been punished for some reason. Parents often blame themselves for in some way causing their child's seizures. Guilt may be a fleeting experience or a lengthy process. The parent may make comments like, "What did I do wrong in the pregnancy?" or "What's wrong with *me?*" or "If I had known, I could have prevented . . ." the accident or the illness, or whatever seems responsible. Release of anger and resolution of feelings of guilt are essential since overindulgence of the child can result from inability to progress through this stage.

Stage V: Depression. Depression is a common and often necessary stage, but may not be recognized by the parents or professional. In this stage, the parents gradually are reconciled to the fact of a seizure disorder and the management necessary. This initially leads the parents into despondency or depression, especially when they realize that the condition may be a lifetime one. A lack of sexual feelings may accompany this stage. Embarrassment may cause withdrawal from social contacts or family isolation, even to subconsciously "hiding" the child. Parents frequently report feelings of estrangement from their friends. They may go about their daily lives automatically and without enthusiasm, perhaps for months. This is where a good friend or a parents' group is important, so that there is involvement with others who have experienced similar problems.

The impact of the condition of epilepsy is overwhelming. Suddenly, the amount of supervision required, the added expense, the loss of social contacts, and uncertainty for the future begin to be fully grasped.

Stage VI: Acceptance. The parents gradually begin to accept and deal with the child realistically. The focus changes from the negative aspects of the seizures to the positive aspects of the child. Parents begin to think of the child first and the handicap second. They now begin to help the child accept and deal with the problems. Acceptance is a peaceful resolution within the parents, allowing for a healthy balance of feelings. It can occur when the parents have gone through the stages, have come to terms emotionally with the reality of epilepsy in their child, and now know they are doing everything appropriate to optimize development in their child.

Some parents progress through these stages in a matter of weeks, others take years. Some parents do not go all the way through the process. Those who remain fixed at any of the earlier stages may begin negatively to alter their attitudes and ways of reacting to their child and to the world. The reactions often reflect the unresolved feelings common to these stages, such as rejection, hostility, withdrawal, overprotection, or depression. The result may be failure to provide a good family environment for the child or total absorption of one parent in the handicapped child to the exclusion of the other children or spouse.

Rapid progress through the stages is possible for parents who become knowledgeable about seizures and who have contact with professionals who recognize parental feelings and guide them with positive steps. Some epilepsy clinics have counselors trained in this process.

Parents of a child with a seizure disorder can help themselves by recognizing that they have these feelings, and that they are normal reactions to the situation. The parents by now realize that these stages were in no way a rejection of their child.

If we were to add a *seventh stage,* it would be that of helping the cause by assisting other parents through these difficult stages. Joining a local EFA group, or PTA, or self-help group can be of considerable help to those who might still be in one of the earlier painful stages. Remember, it is *parents,* not the professionals, who have been responsible for most advances in programs for the handicapped in the past. Many of the special education facilities in our country are primarily the result of parents' group pressures. Classes for the trainable mentally retarded, the deaf, the blind, the orthopedically handicapped, and the educationally handicapped were formed as a result of parents' groups who were interested in helping their children. We hope that you, as parents, have passed successfully through the stages, and that you are now in *Stage VII.*

Why do I still feel frightened by the seizures?

Witnessing the first seizure in one's child is a dramatic and disturbing event for any parent. The initial experience, for a parent who is not too knowledgeable about epilepsy, may well cause a panic reaction. The overwhelming feelings experienced during such a traumatic event may persist and recur at even the thought of the episode. Most parents learn to handle seizures after gaining in knowledge and experience but may still feel anxious when thinking of the possibility of a seizure, or may feel uneasy after one has ended.

With the occurrence of a seizure, parents may fear that the condition is worsening, that the child might be in pain or might injure himself. Injury is not very common, and a convulsion does not indicate that the condition has become more serious. There may be anxieties related to possible embarrassment at having a seizure occur publicly or unexpectedly.

The seizures remind parents of some issues that have not been fully resolved in their thoughts. The seizures make us aware of how helpless we are as parents sometimes. There is nothing that can be done to stop a seizure. Parents who tell themselves they can handle the problems of their child begin to feel they have failed when they can do little beyond protection from injury once a seizure begins. Parents need to remind themselves and tell each other that they are doing the best job of parenting they can and that at times everyone feels insecure and vulnerable.

The seizures also remind parents that something different happens to their child periodically that is not happening to other children. This is a hard fact for all parents fully to accept. Many children have diabetes, cancer, cerebral palsy, and numerous other disorders that are permanent and potentially threatening conditions, but with treatement, emotional support, and love, they are able to lead happy and useful lives.

Many parents we have worked with have been better able to handle their fears and concerns after an opportunity to discuss these issues with a trained professional and with other parents having similar concerns.

Why did this happen to our family?

The answer to this question is an elusive one. Statistically, we know that one family out of about forty will have a child who is mentally retarded and one out of about seventy-five to one hundred will have a child with epilepsy.

For those parents who ask the question from a philosophical or theological perspective, the clergy can be most helpful. Also, the following biblical passages are suggested as sources of support and understanding: Psalm 23, Isaiah 40:26–31 and 61:1–3, Luke 14:27 and 11:5–13, I Peter 1:3–9, I Corinthians 12:12–27, Matthew 11:25–30, Romans 8:16–19 and 24–35.

Roy Rogers and Dale Evans, in their touching little book *Angel*

Unaware, written in the 1950s, felt that they had been selected by God to have a child with Down's Syndrome, in order to make them better people and to enable them to help others. Pearl Buck, in *The Child Who Never Grew,* presented the same view. Many parents feel that being given a trial has helped their growth in wisdom, love, and compassion. Certainly the event can present a great opportunity for service. Many of those making significant contributions in the field are themselves parents of a disabled child.

It is important to note that this question is usually asked only during the parents' initial awareness of the condition. It is seldom asked after they have become members of a local parent group, where they can share their mutual concerns, and begin to offer reassurance and help to other parents.

Our adolescent resents his seizures. What can we do?

Many adolescents tend to deny that they have a seizure disorder. This is the age when social peer groups are vitally important, and when many young people become extremely self-conscious. They want to be like everyone else, and often live in fear that their friends may see them have a seizure. They may make excuses or be defensive if they are not able to drive a car or date like their friends. They may also become upset with the lack of self-control inherent in a seizure and, as a consequence, resent the condition that sets them apart from their peers. One serious problem is that they may stop taking their medication, since this is a reminder that the seizures exist. Inadequate medication makes the condition even worse, tending to increase the seizures and thus resulting in further anger and resentment.

The following suggestions for parents may be helpful in resolving these feelings:

1. Encourage the adolescent to maintain the best physical condition possible. A positive self-concept is easier to maintain when one feels he is in good condition.
2. Carefully monitor the medication. Medical control is essential at all times.

3. A teenager with active epilepsy may lose some friends. Do what you can to convince the adolescent that though some associates do not or will not understand epilepsy, a friendship terminated for this reason was not a valid one to begin with. An adolescent is best prepared to deal with prejudice by having full knowledge of his own epilepsy, strong feelings of self-worth, and the ability to relate well to people.
4. If the seizure disorder will prohibit the adolescent's obtaining a driver's license, prepare him with this fact before the time to take driver's training.
5. Recommend that the adolescent talk freely about the condition to his close friends and encourage them to ask questions about it.
6. Maintain a good relationship with your teenager so that he can talk to you whenever necessary.
7. Ask your doctor or counselor if there is an adolescent with epilepsy among his patients who has made a good adjustment and to whom your teenager can talk.

On occasion the young person's feelings of resentment may continue, in which case professional consultation is needed. Psychological counseling can relieve the emotional problems allowing improved social functioning and better access to the person's own capabilities.

What attitudes do teenagers have toward epilepsy?

In a recent study of the attitudes of adolescents regarding epilepsy, Breger (1976) found that most had heard of epilepsy, but only one third had ever seen a seizure. They were aware that medication could control seizures, but the overwhelming majority thought that seizures would cause death, and almost half believed that persons with epilepsy were violent. Teenagers with accurate information were those who had some personal knowledge of someone with the condition. Most teenagers indicated the condition of epilepsy wouldn't keep them from being friends with someone they liked.

How can we go out? We are unable to get a baby-sitter.

Part of our life-style is for parents to have occasional evenings out together. Not only is this good for the parents, it is also good for children to know that their parents are not always at their beck and call. A baby-sitter and respite care are essential for parents whose child has epilepsy, since it is difficult for parents to cope with the constant care often required. The more severe the child's condition, the greater the need for the parents to have a temporary break from the total care of their child. Mothers as well as fathers often feel trapped, and may begin to resent the child, subconsciously considering it to be the child's fault.

Most parents we know have had to train their own baby-sitters, recognizing that an ordinary baby-sitter is not appropriate for a child with uncontrolled seizures. You should select a mature and responsible person who is willing to learn to provide regular care for your child with seizures. Once a baby-sitter has been trained to recognize the symptoms and to provide the same treatment that you as parents give, there is no need to feel that the child is in any greater danger than if *you* were there.

In a few metropolitan areas, professional baby-sitting services have persons with some experience with seizures and homemaker services may have employees trained in the management of epilepsy. The planned use of respite care allows the whole family to rest for a few days in situations where the child has severe or uncontrolled seizures or constant management problems. Sometimes the services include special nurseries or specialized temporary foster homes for the child who is unable to go on family vacations.

Admittedly, there is a need for more facilities to care for children with epilepsy on a short-term basis, allowing the family time for relaxation.

What family accommodations are advisable for adults with epilepsy?

Family members need to understand the treatment and the first-aid procedures for seizures. It is also important for spouse and friends to be encouraging and supportive as the individual with epilepsy makes necessary personal adjustments. However, it is critical that the person retain responsibility for his or her own life. If help is needed, it should be assistance in performing a task, not assumption of it. The person should not shirk responsibilities because of epilepsy.

Changes in the life-style of an adult with seizures should be minimized in order to maintain optimal functioning. The one major modification often required is that the person must stop driving. Other family members may have to assume this task until it can be determined that it is safe for the person to drive.

7

EDUCATION

What should we as parents tell the school about our child with epilepsy?

First, be sure to let the teachers and school nurse know that your child has epilepsy, even if the child is under good seizure control. Seizures should never be a surprise to the people working with your child. If the youngster has been in special education or will need it, you should also inform the Director of Special Education.

We suggest meeting with the teachers and the nurse to talk about your child so that they may get to know him or her in a personal way and to be totally aware of the condition. Do so in a relaxed manner before any seizures or problems occur. The school nurse should know the type of seizure, the frequency, the medication and dosage, and the name of the physician. Also, the nurse should know whether you wish to be notified about any seizures that occur at school. Moreover, in observing the child at school when the physician is adjusting the medication or dosage, the nurse can assist by providing objective information to the physician of the child's reaction to the change.

Ask the teacher not to give the child any special privileges because of seizures, such as failure to discipline the child when needed, fewer assignments, extra rest periods, and so on. These will only tend to make the child feel "different," and cause the other children to dislike or resent your child. The only exception should be any specific activities prohibited by the physician or the provision of additional help to compensate for a learning disability.

Can the teacher be aware of signs of possible or potential epilepsy in a child?

There is, of course, no difficulty in recognizing a generalized tonic-clonic seizure. However, there are signs which, if repeated, may be used to alert a teacher to the possibility that a child might have epilepsy. If a child has two or more of the following symptoms, and they recur, the teacher might do well to consult the health personnel:

1. Staring spells, or daydreaming
2. Ticlike movements
3. Rhythmic movements of the head
4. Purposeless sounds and body movements
5. Head drooping
6. Lack of response
7. Eyes rolling upward
8. Excessive chewing and swallowing movements

What precautions should the teacher take, knowing that a child is subject to seizures?

The teacher should remember, first of all, that for the child with epilepsy the attitudes of his peers are vitally important. The more normal a school life the child can be permitted to lead, the better his response to medical treatment. This is perhaps the teacher's most important role — providing the child with a normal classroom situation. Normal physical and mental activities tend to have the effect of reducing seizures, and the teacher should avoid overprotecting the child by curbing activities or insisting on rest periods that have not been prescribed. Boredom or frequent rest periods may even result in more seizures than activity or exertion.

Certain precautions, however, should be taken, and activities that need to be closely watched are those in which danger is present should a seizure occur. These would include using power tools, climbing high places, and swimming.

What should the teacher do in the event of a seizure?

Because of the brief nature of petit-mal absence seizures, no action is really necessary. However, should a child have a generalized tonic-clonic (grand mal) or psychomotor attack at school, the teacher will need to handle the situation calmly and instruct the other children to clear the area of sharp objects and not to interrupt the seizure. Nothing should be forced between the teeth. If possible, the teacher should place the student on his side to allow saliva to flow from his mouth. The child will need to rest, perhaps in the nurse's room, following a grand mal seizure. If the child is alert following a seizure, the teacher may have him return to the class and resume the instruction. If the teacher shows a calm, understanding attitude and is encouraging to the child, the other students will quickly come to behave similarly. The students will normally adopt and reflect the attitude and reaction of their teacher, especially at the younger age levels.

If the situation is handled well, the upsetting effect of a convulsion will be transitory and the child will not be regarded as different. When the child is out of the classroom, the teacher should explain to the class that a seizure is a symptom of a problem in the body, that the condition is not contagious, that medication can help, and that the child will not be sick or die. The teacher should instruct them that during any jerking they should allow the child to remain and to remove things which might hurt him, and not try to hold the child still. They need to understand that the child may be sleepy following the seizure but will rejoin them later. The most important thing they can do is to be a friend.

Such an incident, far from being traumatic to the other children, can and should be an excellent learning situation. The teacher should encourage and answer any questions the students have about the episode. The teacher may need to speak privately to the student who rejects or refuses to associate with the epileptic child, or to those who later call him bad names. The teacher should also talk privately with any child who seems upset by having viewed a seizure.

How should teachers treat a child with seizure disorders?

A teacher who is knowledgeable about epilepsy can help the child with seizures cope with the school-related problems so often associated with the disorder. Because of the prejudice and lack of understanding of epilepsy in the general community, a child may feel rejection or sense ridicule by those who see his convulsion. The child soon becomes aware, realistically or unrealistically, of this reaction by his classmates. How the teacher handles the situation will set the tone for how the other children regard the child with seizures. As we have mentioned, the extent to which pupils emulate the attitudes of the teacher, especially at the elementary level, is remarkable.

Restrictions should not be imposed or privileges given because the child has epilepsy. Occasionally, a physician will restrict a child from some body contact sports, but generally no other restrictions on academic, social, or physical activities are necessary. In fact, the more the child participates, the greater his chance for a normal life, and the less the likelihood of seizures.

As a rule, teachers need to treat the child with epilepsy as they would any other child in the classroom.

What should be done if the teacher or school does not seem to understand seizures?

If the teacher or other school staff do not seem knowledgeable about seizures, you must be the one to educate them. Do not assume that the teacher, principal, or other school personnel are necessarily aware of epilepsy. At best, they may have had one or two lectures on the subject during their professional training. Remember, there most probably was a time before your child developed seizures when *you* knew very little about epilepsy. As parents of the child, you are usually better informed than many professionals who have not made a specific study of epilepsy, and you are in an excellent position to provide the knowledge yourselves.

We have found that the best procedure is for you to talk with the school staff about your child, so that they learn of the child as a person. Then ask the teacher or principal if they would like to understand seizure disorders better. If the answer is affirmative, and few educators would be willing to decline, give them this book and the following pamphlets from the EFA: *Epilepsy: The Teacher's Role; Teacher's Tips about the Epilepsies; The Role of the School Nurse in the Understanding and Treatment of Epilepsy.* (These pamphlets are listed in Appendix C.)

We have often suggested that parents go to the trouble and minor expense of purchasing and providing these materials themselves, since the school staff are generally busy and will appreciate the gesture and recognize more readily its importance. The expenditure of a few dollars will be repaid through greater understanding and assistance for your child, as well as for children in general.

If the school staff show continued interest in epilepsy, direct them to the Epilepsy School Alert program described in the next question. This program can aid in further understanding not only by the staff, but by the other children in the school as well.

You might also consider a brief presentation at the school staff or PTA meeting, with a film and discussion. The film *Epilepsy: For Those Who Teach* is excellent for this purpose. It describes what to do if seizures occur in the classroom and promotes understanding of and emotional support for the child with epilepsy. Details regarding the rental of this and other films are included in Appendix D.

What is the School Alert program?

The need for public education about epilepsy is well known. The Commission for the Control of Epilepsy and Its Consequences estimates that currently only about 1 percent of American school children are being reached with literature and information about the disorder.

The Epilepsy Foundation of America is attempting to remedy this by establishing many programs of educating the public as well as the schools about seizure disorders. One of the major programs is School Alert, which has been in successful operation since 1969. In some states (for example, New York and New Hampshire) the School Alert program has been officially endorsed and is operated in direct cooperation with the state departments of education.

The program is essentially educative, designed for local EFA use with the schools in an area. It contains guides for classroom teachers and the school personnel in recognizing and properly managing seizures in the school. School Alert also supplies literature, films, posters, and even lesson plans that can be used. School personnel who are interested in obtaining these materials should contact their local EFA chapter.

Can anticonvulsant medication be given at school?

Yes, if necessary. Most school systems allow for the administration of medication by selected personnel with written permission and instructions by the parent or physician. Normally, the physician writes a note to the school nurse or special education teacher outlining the dosage and schedule of medication. Most school systems then require a consent slip to be signed by the parents.

The medication is kept by the school and is administered according to the prescribed schedule. The medication should never be sent back and forth by the child, nor should it be taken by the child alone. Most districts do not permit the medication to be kept in the teacher's desk, because of the possibility of its accidental use by other children. In one school known to the authors, all the medication was kept in the desk of the school secretary, who had the name of the child, the dosage, and the schedule carefully written on each bottle. The teacher routinely sent the child to the school office at the arranged times, and the school secretary carefully saw to it that the child had the medication, then recorded the time of administration.

There have been unfortunate cases of negligence, and most schools are well aware of the importance of a rigid set of rules regarding medication schedules.

If my child has epilepsy, will he be placed in a special class at school?

Not necessarily, and if so, not because of epilepsy so much as for the conditions that may accompany it. Nearly all children with epilepsy belong in school and most can attend regular, rather than special, classes. The child with epilepsy should be encouraged to lead as normal a life as possible, and this includes attending school with siblings and peers.

Just as other children do, these pupils have the normal wide range of intelligence. The average child with epilepsy falls within the range of normal intelligence; thus, if a child with epilepsy should need to be in a special class for whatever reason, it usually has little to do with epilepsy. Only in a situation in which the child has numerous and prolonged seizures that prevent learning might a special class be required on the basis of epilepsy alone. A child with less frequent seizures, and without other problems, needs to be in a regular classroom.

When the child has gained good seizure control, it is often possible for the physician to remove all restrictions on activities. Though each child must be considered individually, most have been able to participate in athletics, in driver education programs, and in all other phases of school life.

Do children with epilepsy, then, have no problems in school?

The child with epilepsy may well have no difficulties at school. Not all children fare this well, however. The Commission for the Control of Epilepsy and Its Consequences reports that 50 percent of school-age children with epilepsy experience learning difficulties, and that 30 percent have personality or behavioral problems. The child with both a seizure disorder and a behavioral or learning disorder will undoubtedly have difficulty in school.

It has been our experience that many parents often assume that the seizure disorder is the child's only problem, and that an accompanying learning disability is because of the teaching, the loss of instruction during a seizure, or the effects of the child's medication. Problems in learning can occur because of these situations. However, a learning disability may also exist. The learning disability may be caused by the same problems in the brain that produce the seizures. If the disturbance is in a specific area of the brain, it may control the child's ability to process language, read, speak normally, or remember well. Many children with seizures show signs of minimal brain dysfunction in neurological and psychological examinations similar to those in children who do not have epilepsy. These children respond to special education techniques appropriate for learning disabled (LD) students.

What is a learning disability?

A learning disability is a disorder in a child of average intellectual capacity that interferes with the acquisition of basic skills expected of the particular age group. It is associated with impairment of processing in one or more functions of the central nervous system that involve perception, conceptualization, language, memory, or attention. The disorder may show up as a difficulty in listening, thinking, reading, writing, or doing arithmetic. The symptoms are often subtle, but the interference with learning may range from mild to severe. A learning disability does not include problems due to physical conditions such as poor vision or hearing, or side effects of medication, or mental retardation. Some children have mixed conditions, including hyperactivity.

Learning disabilities can occur in association with seizures of any type, but in our experience they are more common with partial seizures, especially those originating in the temporal lobes. Persons with seizure activity in the left temporal areas are prone to learning disabilities involving difficulty in discriminating between similar sounds, in remembering what they have heard, and often in reading. Those with seizures in the right temporal areas may have perceptual-motor difficulties, as in recognizing shapes and orientation of letters and numbers. When writing, such people may reverse letters or words.

Learning disabilities are usually evident in children but may persist into adolescence and adulthood.

How does a child qualify for special education?

Children with epilepsy may qualify under the Education of All Handicapped Children Law 94–142, which provides for special education for physically handicapped students in the section "Other Health Impaired." The "Other Health Impaired" are defined in the law as children with "limited strength, vitality, or alertness due to chronic or acute health problems such as a heart condition, tuberculosis, rheumatic fever, nephritis, asthma, sickle-cell anemia, hemophilia, epilepsy, lead poisoning, leukemia, or diabetes, which adversely affect a child's educational performance."

A child with epilepsy may also have associated problems, such as learning disabilities, social-emotional handicaps, or mental retardation. If the disability requires substantial adaptation of the normal curriculum and instructional techniques, the child may then qualify for special education services. These may be provided within the setting of a regular school.

If your child needs a special class to function at his or her best, then make sure he or she gets into the special education program. As parents, you should not let your own fears or feelings of stigma get in the way of placing your child in the best environment for learning. (The state offices for special education are listed in Appendix A.)

What is the Education of All Handicapped Children Law?

In 1975, the Education of All Handicapped Children Act (PL 94–142) was passed to reorganize special education and to make special education services available to children in every state. It is based on the premise that all American youngsters, without exception, have the right to an education that is free of charge to the parents. The primary goal is to give all handicapped children the learning opportunities they need to be as self-sufficient and productive as possible.

According to current estimates, approximately one half of the nation's eight million handicapped children have been denied the kind of education they need to reach their own potential because of lack of facilities, staff, and techniques. This landmark legislation goes further than any other law to reach these children and change the direction of their lives. In the exact words of the law, its purpose is:

To assure that all handicapped children have available to them a free and appropriate education which emphasizes special education and related services designated to meet their unique needs.

Under this law, states are eligible to participate in the federal plan with federal aid available to pay part of the additional cost of educating handicapped children. The mandatory ages served are three to eighteen, with the upper age limits expanded to twenty-one as of September 1980. The school districts are required to provide trained personnel and programs to meet the needs of each handicapped child or arrange for private special education to meet those needs. The law has permanent authority, with no expiration date.

It is of considerable importance for all parents of handicapped children to know the basic provisions of this law. They are: The highest priority must be given, first, to all handicapped children who are not in school, and second, to the most severely handicapped whose education is inadequate. The law requires an intensive and continuing effort to locate children with handicaps.

The law gives strong consideration to educating children in the "least restrictive environment." It requires children to be placed in special or separate classes only when it is impossible to have a satisfactory placement in a regular classroom with supplementary aids and services because of the nature and severity of the child's handicap. Every effort will be made to continue the handicapped child's contact with his regular classroom, even if only for a portion of the school day. This is based on the principle of "mainstreaming," an educational practice of mixing the handicapped and nonhandicapped together to the maximum extent appropriate.

All methods used for testing and evaluation must be racially and culturally nondiscriminatory and must be administered in the primary language of the child.

Individualized instructional plans are to be prepared for each handicapped child, with the parents participating on the team that develops the plan. These learning prescriptions must include both short- and long-term educational goals and services to be provided.

When handicapped children are placed in private schools by state or local educational systems in order to receive an appropriate education not available in the local public school, this must be done at no cost to the parents. The private school special education program must meet the standards set by law.

The law encourages the development of programs for pre-school-age children. Specific help when the child is young can prevent further handicaps and allow for more rapid growth.

Each state must set up an advisory board that includes handicapped individuals, teachers, and parents of the handicapped. This board is to advise the state on unmet needs and must review the regulations. Local school districts or regions will set up similar advisory boards for their own programs. The duties involve advice, review, and assistance to the educational personnel providing programs for the handicapped.

Strong safeguards of the rights of parents and children are guaranteed under this law. These safeguards protect the parents' rights in all procedures related to identification, evaluation, and placement of their children. Prior written parental consent is required at each stage. The parents shall also have the right and opportunity to examine all relevant school records of their children.

If a parent would like to read the full law (which has been condensed in this question), he or she might contact the special education department of the local or county school district. A copy of this law may also be obtained by writing to your congressman, requesting PL 94–142.

What is IEP?

An "individual educational program" (IEP) is a written, comprehensive plan developed by a team of professionals, and is a method of providing specific educational programming for the child. The plan requires input from all professionals who may be involved in providing for the child's educational services, including the parents, as mandated by PL 94–142. A meeting must be held to discuss the plan, which the parents and in some cases the child, may attend. The meeting should result in priorities for the educational programming, the specific goals to be attained, identification of the persons who will provide the services, and determination of how the program plan will be evaluated.

In preparation for development of the IEP, an assessment must be made of the child's current level of performance in appropriate skill areas. These skill areas involve the following, depending upon the age of the child:

1. Gross-motor — general mobility or ambulation
2. Fine-motor — skilled hand movements, including eye-hand coordination
3. Social — ability to relate appropriately with others
4. Self-help — ability to accomplish tasks of feeding, toileting, dressing, etc.
5. Cognitive — ability to perform academic skills
6. Communicative — ability to receive and express language
7. Recreative — ability to use leisure time
8. Self-concept — ability of a child to feel "good" about himself and his skills
9. Prevocational/vocational — career development
10. Others deemed appropriate

A specific objective or set of objectives will be developed for improving performance in each area. The IEP is simply a statement of the specific learning objectives and the services to be delivered, but is of course not a guarantee that the child will accomplish these objectives. The IEP must be reviewed and/or revised periodically, at least every year, and must consider the following:

1. Specific materials required
2. The type of physical education needed for the child
3. The extent to which the child will participate in the regular education program
4. Short-term objectives
5. The timetable for each objective

Does PL 94–142 provide for services other than classroom instruction?

Under the provisions of PL 94–142, school districts must provide for a number of specialized services to enhance the effectiveness of educational instruction. They include audiology, medical services, occupational therapy, physical therapy, school psychological services, school health services, speech therapy, parent counseling, and transportation. Dependent upon the specific needs of your child, any of the appropriate services listed above can be obtained to assist your child in benefiting fully from special education.

Could a speech therapist be of help?

If your child has a specific speech problem, an evaluation by a speech pathologist is usually warranted. A speech therapist can help with pronunciation and articulation (the way sounds are formed), rhythm, voice control, and language usage. A speech therapist and other professionals will be necessary for special disorders, such as stuttering or aphasia. The services may be available in the public school system or privately. If a speech therapist works with your child, be sure to find out what you can do at home to reinforce the speech therapy the child is receiving.

Can our child with seizures use the school bus?

At one time, this was an area of controversy. Many school districts in the past have required that a child be seizure-free before being permitted to ride the school bus. However, the Education of All Handicapped Children Law includes transportation as a student's "right" to access to education and places the responsibility for transportation on the school district. If for some reason the child is considered unable to ride the regular school bus, he is now generally provided transportation along with other handicapped in a minibus or taxi.

As a regular precaution, it is well to alert the driver of the bus about the possibility of a seizure. The parent has the right to inquire about the training the bus driver received (including handling seizures), to ask about seat belts, and to suggest that a buddy system be used.

If the child has sufficient seizure control to attend school, he should then be able to use the specialized school transportation system. Of course, if the seizures are well controlled, the child can and should ride the regular school bus.

Can my child attend the Head Start program?

Project Head Start began as a demonstration program in 1964 to provide health, social, and educational services to disadvantaged preschool children. In 1976 the eligibility was changed to require that 10 percent of all children enrolled be handicapped. As a result, many children with epilepsy can now attend Head Start. Epilepsy is included in the definition of handicap under "Health or Developmental Impairments," with the phrase "Developmental Impairments" referring to illnesses of a chronic nature with prolonged convalescence. This includes epilepsy and other neurological disorders.

To be eligible, handicapped children must be between the age of three and the age of compulsory school attendance in the state of residence. Most programs provide services during the years immediately prior to entrance into public school. Not all handicapped children are required to be from low-income families. Many parents who may not qualify under the classification of "low income" have not been aware of the mandatory 10 percent handicapped provision and as a result have failed to take advantage of Head Start.

Head Start provides a comprehensive program of educational, psychological, dental, and nutritional services. Medical services, speech therapy, and specialized consultation are available for a child as needed. Parents are encouraged to participate in the program and to attend parents' meetings. It has been our experience that the Head Start programs are of high quality, providing a clear advantage to those children enrolled, in both skill development and confidence.

For information about the program and your child's eligibility, check the telephone directory or contact the local public school district for the Head Start program in your area.

Are vocational education programs available at schools?

Programs are increasingly available in both high schools and adult schools throughout the nation. One major program is funded by matching grants from Title II of the 1976 amendments to the Vocational Education Act. Local schools or cooperative school districts can operate such programs for the handicapped; in fact, by law 10 percent of each state grant for vocational education *must* be used for these special programs. The term "handicapped" includes "mentally retarded and other health impaired," including those with epilepsy, who because of their condition cannot succeed in the regular vocational program without special assistance. The programs are designed to provide a wide range of vocational training, work-study, and placement services for those who finish the programs.

The regular vocational education programs are available for individuals not requiring services for the handicapped. Most programs provide individualized and practical training and job experience in a variety of occupations deemed to have a shortage of trained personnel in the community. Programs are available for both high school students and adults. Contact the local vocational training center or high school for information.

How can the school help with vocational preparation?

Teachers and high school counselors can assist the student with epilepsy in the selection and preparation of an appropriate education that is compatible with the disability. Of course, persons with seizures must realize that certain occupations (such as commercial airline pilot, truck driver, surgeon, baby-sitter, telephone line repairman, and so forth) are not appropriate. Certain national security positions should also be avoided. However, there are far more positions available than the handful that are not.

For the child having seizures during junior or senior high school, it should be considered possible that the seizures may continue, and he should prepare for an occupation that will allow for the disorder. A disappointment early is better than a disaster later. The student with epilepsy faces a good likelihood of restrictions in future employment. Even when seizures are controlled, he must realize that a lack of understanding on the part of many employers will be encountered in obtaining employment. The best assurances of employment are for the student (1) to make an appropriate vocational choice in the beginning, and (2) to prepare himself so well that his skill and training overcompensate for any handicap the epilepsy may present.

In prevocational guidance, the teacher, counselor, and parent must work together. They will need information from the physician regarding the expected seizure pattern for adulthood. An examination by the psychologist is necessary to delineate the student's vocational aptitudes, interests, and ability level. The student should then select an occupation that fits his interests, aptitudes, capabilities, and projected demand in the competitive employment market. A student should be guided to select an occupation that is not overcrowded, is not declining, uses his talents, and requires specialized training.

What is the best means of predicting academic success?

The measure of overall intelligence (IQ), based on an individual rather than a group intelligence test, is the best single predictor of academic success, though it is of course no guarantee. Many factors, such as the child's motivation, self-concept, seizure frequency, ability to concentrate, listening skills, friendship patterns, interest in school, parental encouragement, and the learning environment, make up the other major variables. All of these, taken together, can give a good prediction of success in school tasks.

8

HELPING AGENCIES

What is a developmental disability?

A developmental disability has been defined as a severe disability that is due to mental retardation, cerebral palsy, epilepsy, autism, or other neurological disorders that result in a similar impairment of intellectual and/or adaptive social development. This definition has recently been modified by Public Law 95–602 (November 1978) through amendments to the original Developmental Disabilities Act of 1971. The definition now reads as follows:

The term "Developmental Disability" means a severe chronic disability of a person which —

a. is attributable to a mental or physical impairment or combination of mental and physical impairments;
b. is manifested before the person attains age twenty-two;
c. is likely to continue indefinitely;
d. results in substantial functional limitations in three or more of the following areas of major life activity: (i) self-care, (ii) receptive and expressive language, (iii) learning, (iv) mobility, (v) self-direction, (vi) capacity for independent living, and (vii) economic sufficiency; and

e. reflects the person's need for a combination and sequence of special, interdisciplinary, or generic care, treatment, or other services which are of lifelong or extended duration and are individually planned and coordinated.

In the terms of this definition, some persons with epilepsy qualify as developmentally disabled if the epilepsy appears before the age of twenty-two and is a substantial handicap to the individual. Primarily, those persons whose seizures are not well controlled or whose seizures interfere with three or more of the major life areas mentioned above, so that they are unable to profit from normal activities expected at their age, qualify as having major limitations. One's eligibility for services as a developmentally disabled person, then, is based on the presence of a chronic disability that results in substantial functional limitations.

What does the federal government provide for the developmentally disabled?

Many laws have been passed by the federal government to assist in the planning and delivery of services to handicapped people. Landmark legislation includes the Mental Retardation Facilities and Community Mental Health Center Construction Act of 1963 (PL 88–164); the Developmental Disabilities Services and Facilities Amendments of 1970 (PL 91–517); the Developmentally Disabled Assistance and Bill of Rights Act of 1975 (PL 94–103); and the amendments to that act of 1978 (PL 95–602). Many other federal laws affect the handicapped, as well.

In general, the overall purpose of these acts is to "assist the states to assure that persons with developmental disabilities receive the care and treatment necessary to enable them to achieve their maximum potential." This purpose is realized through assistance to the states in appropriate planning activities and through grants to the states and to public and private nonprofit agencies for the establishment of model programs, demonstration of new techniques, and training of professional personnel. Since the provisions of the laws are carried out through the states, their scope varies from state to state. In general, each state may prepare a plan that will enable it to receive a federal allocation, matched by state funds, that must be spent on the objectives in that plan. The plan may involve contracts with agencies or may provide grants to local agencies or hospitals, for some or all of the following services: diagnosis, evaluation, treatment, personal care, day care, domiciliary care, special living arrangements, training, education, sheltered employment, recreation, counseling of the disabled person and family, referral and information services, transportation.

Many of these services can be obtained at a center for the developmentally disabled, sometimes one combined with the Comprehensive Mental Health Centers discussed in the next answer. These centers for the developmentally disabled are not, however, found nationwide, and in some areas the services are very limited. To find out what is available in your area, check the telephone book for the agency that serves the developmentally disabled. If you are unable to find it, contact the health department or the office of developmental disabilities in your state (listed in Appendix A).

What services are available in a Comprehensive Mental Health Center (CMHC)?

These centers provide mental health care for all persons in the community. In some areas the services for mental health and for developmental disabilities are combined in a Comprehensive Mental Health and Mental Retardation Center. Such centers are available throughout the country, providing services on a 24-hour basis.

Under contract with the federal government, the centers must provide basic services, including hospitalization for psychiatric problems, partial hospitalization that involves intensive treatment while allowing the person to live at home, emergency services, outpatient diagnosis and treatment, services to children, special problems of the elderly, and services related to alcohol or drug problems. Persons with epilepsy who have difficulty coping with daily living, show extreme or sudden changes in behavior, or need help with emotional problems are eligible for these services

All residents living in the area served by the CMHC are eligible to receive needed services. The cost is determined on a sliding scale, depending on the ability to pay.

What is Title XX of the Social Security Act?

The Social Security Act, Title XX — usually referred to simply as "Title Twenty" — makes available through the states a wide range of social services to low-income families or individuals. These services are provided by the staffs of public agencies or by contracts with private providers. States may choose what services they may offer, including adoption, counseling, case management, referral, day care, homemaker services, and others. The program also provides funds for training of personnel in a service facility. Some of these services may be relevant to people with seizure disorders and their families.

The services must be directed toward the most appropriate of the following goals: self-support, self-sufficiency, protection, community care, and institutional care.

Although Title Twenty is part of the Social Security Act, it is adr.. istered on the state level. To find out more about its provisions, contact the local Social Service agency or the state department of public welfare.

What is SSI?

The Supplemental Security Income (SSI) program is a federal cash-benefit program for elderly, blind, or disabled persons who need added income to meet their basic living needs of food, clothing, and shelter. It is a way of compensating for the added expense of a disability.

The SSI program is administered by the Social Security Administration. The eligibility and benefits are similar in all fifty states and the District of Columbia. A welfare program is maintained in Guam, Puerto Rico, and the Virgin Islands. Besides the federal SSI benefit, some states provide additional monies in the form of a state supplement.

How does a disabled person qualify for SSI benefits?

To qualify for SSI a person must meet the definition of "disabled," be in need of finances for providing basic needs, meet the residency requirements, and have limited resources. Some individuals may receive partial benefits if their financial condition does not warrant full payments.

For a person to qualify as disabled with a convulsive disorder, documentation of the epilepsy is necessary. This will require an accurate and detailed description of the seizures, preferably as observed by a physician, and substantiated by an EEG tracing. Determination of the disability will be made on the basis of the severity of the epilepsy. The general guideline allows for major motor seizures occurring more than once each month with treatment, and minor motor seizures occurring more frequently than once each week with treatment. Individuals with multiple impairments, such as mental retardation combined with epilepsy, may qualify even with less severe impairments, because of the combination of conditions.

Eligibility for adults differs somewhat from that for children who are disabled. An adult must have a physical or mental impairment, prior to the age of eighteen, that may be expected to last at least one year and that keeps the person from working. A child must have a physical or mental impairment that may be expected to continue and that hampers the child's growth and development.

Besides the benefits from the SSI program, qualification is also important since it makes one automatically eligible for Medicaid in most states.

How does one apply for SSI benefits?

Any individual may apply if he considers himself or his child eligible for benefits. The Social Security office will evaluate the situation and determine eligibility.

One may obtain an application form by writing, calling, or visiting any Social Security office. The Social Security Administration maintains service offices in most areas of the country. The location of the nearest office can be found in the telephone book under United States Government, Health and Human Services Department, Social Security Administration.

An application is considered completed when the application form is filled in, signed by the "claimant" (the disabled person who would receive benefits), and returned to the Social Security office. A parent may apply on behalf of his child. The application may be returned by mail, but there is an advantage if it is returned in person, since an interview is often necessary. The applicant should take with him a copy of his birth certificate and the names and addresses of any specialists who can verify the claimant's condition.

Once an individual is found to be eligible, the Social Security office will generally redetermine financial eligibility and reevaluate the severity of the condition periodically. Any substantial change in the disability should be reported to the Social Security office. Should the application be denied, the determination may be appealed.

For children or severely disabled persons, a "representative payee" may be appointed. This is a person, such as a parent or guardian, who receives the payment and uses the money to provide for the basic personal needs of the disabled person.

The SSI benefits vary by state depending upon whether the state adds money to the basic federal payment. At present, thirty-eight states provide such supplements.

The Social Security office will determine the monthly payment based on the living arrangement of the adult or child and the individual financial need. For example, the basic monthly federal payment for an adult or child is at present $264.70. The total payment will be higher in states that add supplements, and decreased if the individual has other income. For a child residing with the parents the payment will be reduced in relation to the income of the family. Children who require residential care apart from the family receive the full monthly payment plus any state supplement for the living cost. For individuals requiring private hospitalization the SSI payment is reduced to $25 per month for personal needs, with Medicaid covering the hospital costs.

What is Medicaid?

Medicaid (MediCal in California) is an important source of assistance for health care to low-income families. People of low income who have a child with epilepsy, and therefore more medical bills, can benefit substantially from the program. The Medicaid program is available in all states except Arizona and in the District of Columbia, Guam, Puerto Rico, and the Virgin Islands.

The Medicaid program was enacted as part of the Social Security Act in 1965 to assist states in providing health care costs for those with low income. Under the program, eligible adults or children with epilepsy can obtain a Medicaid card and have the bills paid by the state and federal governments. The card is issued for each eligible person and cannot be used by anyone else. The coverage includes physician, psychologist, clinic, hospital, laboratory and X-ray, skilled nursing-home, and family planning services. Children covered under Medicaid can use the prevention and medical screening services of Early and Periodic Screening, Diagnosis, and Treatment (EPSDT). Most states pay for prescription drugs. Some states also cover necessary long-term institutionalization or group-home treatment for the developmentally disabled under Medicaid.

Persons of low income eligible for welfare and cash assistance are automatically eligible to receive Medicaid coverage. Children receiving SSI for a disability are eligible for Medicaid in most states. Some states also allow families who earn slightly more than the financial maximum for welfare but have family members who are "medically needy" to obtain only the Medicaid card.

To apply for the Medicaid card, contact the welfare department or health department operating the program in your area.

Are there any veterans' benefits for persons with epilepsy?

Many of the veterans' hospitals have neurology services capable of providing medical care for veterans with epilepsy. Seven of these hospitals have Epilepsy Centers designed for specialized treatment of complex cases. Veterans may be transferred to these centers if necessary. All United States veterans are eligible for services unless they received dishonorable discharges. For specific services, call the nearest VA hospital.

What services can Crippled Children's Services provide? Do children with epilepsy qualify?

Children who have severe physically handicapping conditions that require extensive or expensive treatment are eligible for Crippled Children's Services (CCS), administered by the state departments of public health. The eligibility includes persons under the age of twenty-one with severe and/or uncontrolled seizures. The program can provide financial assistance to help families obtain comprehensive treatment or, in some states, can provide direct treatment, including diagnostic treatment and medication. Most states require the parents to pay a portion of the costs of service. Some may offer follow-up services until the seizure condition is under control and the family has passed the period of heavy financial burden.

Each state has its own plan for the provision of services. Some states do not include the word "crippled" in the name of the program but use such titles as Handicapped Children's Services or Child Health Services. For the program in your area, contact the appropriate state office on the list in Appendix A.

What services do the departments of vocational rehabilitation provide?

Under the Rehabilitation Act of 1973, the state departments of vocational rehabilitation provide services for certain physically and developmentally disabled adults. Persons with convulsive disorders may qualify if it is determined that there is a "reasonable expectation" that the services may lessen the handicaps and enable employment. The state vocational rehabilitation agency can assist individuals over age eighteen with epilepsy to develop vocational skills "appropriate to their potential."

Persons who develop severe seizures *after* they have worked often need retraining because of the disability or danger present in the work. Each state maintains an office of vocational rehabilitation that can provide these services or can help to prepare one with epilepsy for initial employment. The services include assessment of aptitudes and skills, counseling, work evaluations, work adjustment, specialized training, transportation, and placement services. Necessary seizure control procedures may be accomplished to allow the individual to attain optimal benefit from the training program. A vocational plan will be established to determine the type of employment for which the person is best suited. In some cases, the agency has helped persons with epilepsy start small businesses. Basic equipment necessary to establish the business is sometimes provided upon successful completion of the training program.

Persons with epilepsy are considered eligible once the disability has been determined to constitute a "substantial handicap" to employment and their rehabilitation potential has been established. Neurological disorders, including epilepsy, are included under the section of "severely handicapped" as disabilities receiving priority. Applications for services should be made in person at the local office of the state department of vocational rehabilitation.

Are other training and employment programs available?

The employment and vocational training prospects continue to show improvement. Some programs are oriented specifically for persons with epilepsy. One organization of this type that has been most successful is a nonprofit group known as EPI-HAB, standing for Epileptic Rehabilitation. The EPI-HAB companies provide employment and specific training for persons with epilepsy who have difficulty finding employment, yet have industrial skills. The companies have demonstrated that persons with epilepsy can be capable and beneficial employees, with an excellent safety record. The companies are actually mini-industries that contract for work in such areas as packaging, electronics, machine shop, and assembly jobs. Many persons acquire the skill, training, confidence, and experience at EPI-HAB that enable them to obtain employment in the competitive job market.

The EPI-HAB programs operate independently as separate companies, each with its own board of directors. Companies are located in the following cities:

1. EPI-HAB Los Angeles
   5601 South Western Avenue
   Los Angeles, California 90062
2. EPI-HAB Phoenix, Inc.
   2125 West Fillmore
   Phoenix, Arizona 85009
3. EPI-HAB
   201 North Seventh Avenue
   Evansville, Indiana 47710

The first EPI-HAB program was started at the Veteran's Hospital in Los Angeles. Similar programs are maintained in the rehabilitation centers in various veterans' hospitals, notably Los Angeles and Long Island, for veterans with epilepsy.

A program called TAPS (Training and Placement Service) has been developed by the EFA through a contract with the U.S. Department of Labor to provide job training and job placement for those with epilepsy. The centers are located in Atlanta, Boston, Cleveland, Minneapolis/St. Paul, Portland, and San Antonio. Similar programs have been developed in other communities, including Duluth, Minnesota, Savannah, Georgia, Portland, Maine, and Baltimore, Maryland, under funding from vocational rehabilitation and developmental disability grants. It is possible that other cities may soon be added.

The program is new, but may develop into a nationwide resource for young adults having difficulty obtaining skills in job placement due to epilepsy. The program has already been successful in locating jobs for many persons previously unable to find employment.

Teenagers and young adults with seizures under reasonable control may find the federally supported CETA (Comprehensive Employment and Training Act) program a good resource. CETA was started to provide training and generate employment for economically disadvantaged, unemployed, or underemployed persons. To be eligible, a person must be from a low-income family, live in an area of substantial unemployment, or be unemployed within a specific area. No special program is designated for the handicapped, but persons with seizure disorders are included in CETA provisions.

CETA's grants from the Department of Labor are provided to

municipal government to fund sponsors such as schools and private organizations. One of the authors of this book was directly involved in a CETA program and found it to be most helpful in supplying employment opportunities for those who were otherwise not employable. Check the telephone book under government listings for the CETA number in your area. One should be aware that the funding levels for this program have recently been reduced.

What is a sheltered workshop?

A sheltered workshop is a setting in which a handicapped person can learn and work in a protective environment under supervision. Such workshops range from small, part-time programs run by parents or volunteers to large industries operated by professionals. They may be partially supported by the state department of vocational rehabilitation, but more often are financially dependent upon tuition funds, grants, or work subcontracts from local community industry, or placement funds from agencies serving the handicapped.

Workshops offer two types of programs: (1) training, supervision, and work experience for persons who will later leave for regular employment in the competitive job market in the community; and (2) training and continued employment at the workshop in a protective environment. The latter becomes a permanent work placement.

Many handicapped individuals with epilepsy can benefit from the comprehensive training programs and sheltered settings with a supervisor trained and willing to be understanding of a person with seizures. The personnel are also better able to deal with frustrations and self-defeating attitudes frequently experienced by persons with seizure disorders. The goal is to make the person productive. Handicapped individuals eighteen years old and over can apply to enter a workshop.

We have found that young persons with epilepsy often feel more at home in the training program for the handicapped. It is not as intimidating or frightening as competitive employment, and the people do not feel "alone." For those persons with multiple handicaps, such as epilepsy and mild mental retardation or cerebral palsy, the center may offer continued employment not available otherwise.

Most workshops pay wages based on individual productivity. The rate is generally calculated for each individual employee, based on the amount and quality of work produced as compared to normal industrial standards. Even if the rate is low, which it usually is, the worker earns money and gains personal worth as an employee.

Sheltered workshops offer advantages to certain persons with epilepsy, such as those with uncontrolled seizures, the multihandicapped, those needing vocational training, and those who will always require a protective work setting. The advantages to the individual are feelings of personal worth, simulated normal work experiences, vocational training, lasting friendships, money, and the development of good work habits and attitudes. Many of the workshops sponsor social events such as dances, movies, and other recreation for their workers.

Industries are discovering that a number of routine assembly, packaging, labeling, sorting, and repetitive but delicate jobs can be handled better and at a lower cost in a sheltered workshop than in their own plant.

Is assistance available for independent living or supervised living arrangements?

In some areas, rent subsidies are available for eligible, low-income, handicapped persons. Some special-interest loans are also being given for construction of housing for the handicapped. Both programs make community or independent living more accessible for the young adult with seizures.

To qualify for independent-living rent subsidies under Section 8 of the Housing and Community Development Act of 1974, a person with epilepsy must have a family income that does not exceed 80 percent of the middle income of the area. The family may be two or more single handicapped individuals living together, or one handicapped person with an attendant. To participate, a handicapped person should obtain a certificate from the local housing authority, select the housing desired (or available), and have it approved by the housing authority.

There is still a great need for more community semi-independent living facilities for persons with epilepsy. Often, the young person leaving home needs assistance with money management, purchasing, and self-care. Two types of facilities that have been successful are:

1. Group homes. A staff person supervises the home and assists the residents in social and self-help skills necessary for semi-independent living. The degree of supervision can be varied, according to the functioning level of the individual.

2. Semi-independent apartments. These are apartments for one or more individuals, with minimal supervision and assistance.

I need help in the home. What are homemaker services?

Homemaker services provide specially trained persons with skills in homemaking and care of the disabled. Such individuals may be necessary to help with household duties while other family members deal with the epileptic child. They may also be used to provide baby-sitting for the epileptic child to allow the parents an opportunity for necessary recreational and social activities, and also for temporary relaxation from the responsibility of the care of the child. Parents find they are better able to cope with their problems when they have occasional respite from the situation. Remember that raising a child with a serious seizure disorder is often stressful for the entire family.

Homemaker services may be obtained from the social services department of the county or city government or occasionally through private agencies. The parent should ask for a homemaker specially trained to handle epileptic seizures.

What services are available through Easter Seal programs?

One of the largest voluntary agencies providing services to the handicapped is the National Easter Seal Society for Crippled Children and Adults. The organization has chapters throughout the

United States and Puerto Rico. Many volunteers assist the professional staff in providing direct services, as well as fund-raising and transportation.

The programs involve speech therapy, special education programs, handicapped camping, family counseling, and referral services. The national society also supports research, and maintains an advocate role in federal legislation. Check the local telephone directory in your area or contact the national organization.

What are the advantages of membership in the Epilepsy Foundation of America? How do we join?

One can join through either a local chapter or the national office (EFA, 4351 Garden City Drive, Landover, Maryland 20785). A membership costs $12 per year, with part of the funds returned to the local chapter. As a member, you will receive the monthly newsletter, *The National Spokesman*, which is informative for both laymen and professionals. With membership one is also eligible for discounts on prescription medicine and may be eligible for life insurance at group rates.

The EFA acts as an epilepsy information source and an advocate for persons with epilepsy in national programs and in government agencies. It was largely through the efforts of the EFA that valproic acid was recently approved for use in the United States. State and local chapters assist with referrals and public education, and offer an opportunity to meet other persons with similar concerns. The state chapters or information contacts are listed in Appendix A.

What are the new "Comprehensive Epilepsy Programs"?

The National Institute of Neurological and Communicative Disorders and Stroke has selected six centers for demonstration programs of the multidisciplinary concept in delivery of services for persons with epilepsy. The Comprehensive Epilepsy Programs are federally funded and offer total diagnostic, treatment, and counseling services for both patients and family. They are staffed by an interdisciplinary team including a neurologist, psychologist, counselor, speech pathologist, nurse, vocational rehabilitation counselor, and other support staff. The programs provide assistance with follow-up and consultative services. Each center is involved in research regarding services for epilepsy.

The Comprehensive Epilepsy Programs are located at the following facilities:

1. California Comprehensive Epilepsy Program
   Department of Neurology UCLA Center for Health Control
   Los Angeles, California 90024 (213) 824-4303
2. Georgia Comprehensive Epilepsy Program
   Department of Neurology, Medical College of Georgia
   Augusta, Georgia 30901 (404) 828-4533
3. Comprehensive Epilepsy Program
   University of Minnesota School of Medicine
   2829 University Avenue, S.E., Suite 608
   Minneapolis, Minnesota 55414 (612) 376-5031
4. Epilepsy Center of Oregon
   Good Samaritan Hospital and Medical Center
   2222 N.W. Lovejoy, Suite 361
   Portland, Oregon 97210 (503) 229-7220
5. Comprehensive Epilepsy Program
   University of Virginia Medical Center, Box 403
   Charlottesville, Virginia 22901 (804) 924-5401
6. Epilepsy Center at Harborview
   University of Washington School of Medicine
   325 Ninth Avenue
   Seattle, Washington 98104 (206) 233-3573

The programs serve as models for research in neurological disorders and health service delivery methods in epilepsy. They also include educational components for professionals, students and the general public.

What is the Comprehensive Epilepsy Services Network?

The Commission for the Control of Epilepsy and Its Consequences has made an important recommendation for the Nationwide Plan to include a vast network of services to those with epilepsy. This recommendation is considered the most dramatic and innovative ever proposed. The Comprehensive Epilepsy Services Network (CESN) proposes to coordinate the efforts of existing community services, community resource persons, and resource teams, under a Federal Office for Special Neurological Impairments.

It is the hope that this network will maximize the use of existing services at the national level, and markedly reduce seizure problems. The proposed network is discussed in greater detail in the Epilogue.

9

INSURANCE

Does the person with epilepsy have difficulty obtaining insurance?

Obtaining insurance and at a reasonable rate remains a major problem for most persons with epilepsy. Insurance companies have made extensive investigations into the possible risks involved with those they insure. Unfortunately, most of these companies are using obsolete data about epilepsy, with the result that the person with epilepsy, if he *can* get insurance, must usually pay a higher premium. Some insurance companies still use material from the 1929 *Medical Impairment Study*. This study reported a mortality rate for those with epilepsy nearly two and one half times that of the "standard risk" rate. Like this study, most of the others related to mortality and accident risks were done before the discovery and widespread clinical use of the current effective anticonvulsant medications.

Insurance companies view epilepsy as a special risk along with other chronic handicaps. However, it is encouraging to see an increased number of companies adopting a practice of assessing applications from persons with epilepsy on an individual basis rather than relying on outdated statistical information or making a decision based only on a person's belonging to the broad category of epilepsy. While it is true that some persons with epilepsy represent an increased insurance risk, certainly all do not.

Several companies, notably Prudential and Bankers Life and Casualty, have recently reviewed their rules on the basis of their claims experience with persons with epilepsy. They found the results did not warrant as many exclusions and allowed a reduction in the additional premium rates. They have announced changes in underwriting practices that would offer insurance to individuals previously considered ineligible and increase benefits to those already insured.

There are several basic considerations taken into account by insurance companies in evaluating applications. Most companies check for compliance with medical treatment and for frequency of seizures. If the applicant's seizures are controlled medically, the person is more likely to obtain coverage than if he or she is not seizure-free. Companies also check for any complicating medical or physical condition. Employment is often a criterion for acceptance, and unemployed persons will have much greater difficulty obtaining health insurance, in particular. Those with epilepsy who use alcohol or have poor driving records are considered unsatisfactory candidates for insurance.

It is essential that you check with several insurance companies and compare the value of policies, since both price and coverage vary widely. Also, do not assume that if one company rejects an application all companies will do the same. If an agent rejects the application verbally, ask for the reason in writing. This forces the company to take a more careful look at the application and gives you the opportunity to respond, describing your own circumstances.

Since there are so many different insurance companies and the insurance regulations vary by state, it is very difficult to present a meaningful summary that is applicable nationwide. However, this chapter can assist in providing basic information and general guidelines for persons faced with obtaining insurance.

What types of insurance are there?

The major types of insurance of importance to persons with epilepsy are life, health, automobile, and disability insurance.

1. *Life Insurance.* Most persons with epilepsy can obtain life insurance, but because of the limited current data the insurance companies have, the person must usually waive any disability income benefit, as well as pay a higher premium. Some companies determine the premium rate depending on the type of epilepsy, the person's medical history, and the time lapse since the last seizure. The availability of life insurance for those with tonic-clonic seizures is more restricted than for those with absence seizures. Though there is a wide variation in the rates of the various companies, policies are all expensive when one has epilepsy, and it is wiser for the person to obtain group life insurance when possible.

2. *Health Insurance.* The lack of current data also makes it difficult for one with epilepsy to obtain health insurance. Some companies will issue "substandard" health insurance, which waives coverage in cases of disability resulting from or related to epilepsy. In many cases, the person will be restricted as to the type of coverage. Most companies will not offer long-term disability coverage to a person with epilepsy, except for those having the "mildest" forms. Health coverage is usually available (at double the normal premium price) for those with epilepsy who can demonstrate a seizure-free period of several years. As in the case of life insurance, it is better if the person can obtain group health insurance.

3. *Auto Insurance.* Auto insurance is often the most difficult type of coverage for the person with epilepsy to obtain. One must often be refused by from one to three separate companies (according to the state of residence) in order to obtain insurance through an "assigned risk" policy (see page 176).

4. *Disability Insurance.* Several forms of disability insurance are available. They provide money for persons who become disabled and cannot work.

Many authorities feel, and the authors of this book agree, that discrimination against those with epilepsy is unfair, and that it is based on antiquated data. In support of this attitude, Perlman and Strudler (1975) made the following statement:

All it will take . . . is for *one* insurance company to become interested enough in the disorder of epilepsy to take the same time and effort that they have spent on big-name diseases, and do the same for epilepsy. It is time for the truth to be known about the disorder of epilepsy.

These categories of coverage are discussed further in subsequent questions in this chapter.

What about life insurance?

There are two types of life insurance policies — "whole life" and "term life." Whole life is a policy that pays upon death but also maintains a cash value and eventually returns much of the money invested.

Term insurance provides protection but does not have a cash value except upon the death of the insured. Because no savings investment is involved, the premiums are lower than those for whole life policies.

What are "substandard" groups in life insurance?

Individual life insurance policies generally require a physical examination to determine whether the applicant represents a special risk to the company. If the applicant's general health and medical history show problems that represent a higher than average mortality potential, the person is considered from an insurance position as "substandard." Approximately one in every ten applicants for individual life insurance falls into this category and must pay a higher premium. This does not mean that the particular applicant is not expected to live a full life; rather, that certain conditions, as a group, on a purely statistical basis represent a greater risk. Most persons with epilepsy are considered by insurance companies to fall into this substandard group, and the premium rates vary according to the person's individual history. (The substandard consideration also affects health insurance; see page 173.)

The rates usually vary according to the type of seizures, the length of time the person has been seizure-free, the age at which the first seizure occurred, and the person's age.

Insurance companies generally approve applicants whose seizures began in childhood and decreased through the years. The companies do not generally approve applicants with epilepsy who are in their teens, because of the difficulty in reliably "predicting" the severity of seizures in the future.

The EFA has prepared some excellent pamphlets and monographs regarding insurance for persons with epilepsy, which are listed in Appendix C.

Is there currently a group life insurance policy available for persons with epilepsy?

One of the healthiest steps in this direction has recently been taken by the Epilepsy Foundation of America, when it made available a Group Life Insurance Plan for all EFA members. Under this plan, spouses and/or children may also be included. This is term insurance, which specifies a term of coverage and therefore permits lower premium rates. This plan recognizes what many insurance companies do *not*, namely, that most people with epilepsy are not a poor risk for life insurance.

The plan is underwritten by the Government Employees Life Insurance Company (Washington, D.C.), and is available for those who have epilepsy as well as those who do not. Current coverage is from $5,000 to $50,000 for eligible EFA members, ages eighteen through fifty-nine. Once a member is covered under this plan, the protection may be kept on a term renewal basis until age sixty-five; when terminated, it may be converted to a permanent policy. The premiums are waived if the person insured becomes totally disabled before age sixty. The EFA has prepared a free brochure regarding this plan, which is available upon request.

What types of health coverage are available?

There are several basic forms of health insurance, and an individual policy may combine some of the more common types:

1. *Hospital insurance:* the most popular form of health insurance, with four out of five persons in the general population having such protection. It is usually limited to nonoccupational injuries and illnesses.
2. *Surgical insurance:* limited to a maximum amount specified in the policy.
3. *Regular medical expense insurance.*
4. *Major medical expense insurance:* for major illnesses or injuries, usually with a deductible ranging from $50 to $500.

Is individual health insurance available to one with epilepsy?

The differences among insurance companies are so great that it is difficult to make blanket statements. Most insurance companies do not issue individual major medical insurance to persons with epilepsy, and those that do usually provide the coverage on a strictly individual basis for limited periods of time. They are usually reluctant to issue noncancelable policies, even on a substandard basis.

Some companies will consider individual applications when there is a waiting period of up to several months before the policy benefits take effect. The individual is offered "deductible rates," meaning that questionable claims and many small claims are generally not submitted. For these reasons, it is usually recommended that a person with epilepsy has a better chance asking for a waiting period when applying for disability income coverage and for a "deductible" when seeking medical expense coverage.

Often companies will exclude coverage for certain expenses related to epilepsy for a period of time while granting the remainder of the health insurance. These exclusions come under "pre-existing conditions" clauses in the policy.

Obviously, health insurance is more easily obtained when the seizures are medically controlled. If additional physical complications are present, the person is usually placed in a higher premium class or denied coverage altogether.

Some insurance companies also consider the psychological adjustment of the person to epilepsy, and have been known to deny coverage to a person whose seizures are controlled, but who has made an inadequate adjustment to the condition. Many companies also hesitate to underwrite persons with epilepsy who have had difficulties maintaining employment.

It is well to check with a prospective health insurance company about acceptance of a person with epilepsy before changing any group insurance policy. As a general rule, it is better to keep a policy that was in effect and covered the person before epilepsy was diagnosed, even if it means higher premiums.

Are group health insurance plans available for persons with epilepsy?

Group health plans remain the best means of health coverage for persons with epilepsy, since many would be unable to pay for the more expensive individual substandard coverage. The determination of the cost, however, is vastly more complicated than in life insurance, and, unfortunately, most insurance companies still use the same outdated statistics used for life insurance.

Group health insurance offers several obvious advantages to a person with epilepsy, the most important being that it is more easily obtained. Also, the claim rates for group major medical insurance for one with epilepsy are only slightly higher than average, resulting in only a minimal cost to the employer. Studies have shown that employees with epilepsy actually have fewer accidents than other employees. A major advantage is that *none* of the group health coverages excludes persons with epilepsy from hospital or medical coverage.

In 1976, Minnesota enacted legislation to make available health insurance coverage to all persons who had been unable to obtain standard coverage (the Minnesota Comprehensive Health Insurance Act), providing for a pool of insurance companies to help in the problem. It is hoped that this law, which went into effect in January of 1977, will serve as a basis for model legislation in other states, and that it will prove to be a means by which the discriminatory practices toward persons with epilepsy can be reduced.

Can a person with epilepsy join a Health Maintenance Organization?

As an alternative to regular health insurance, a Health Maintenance Organization (HMO) can be a means for persons with epilepsy to obtain health coverage, if one exists in the area. Health Maintenance Organizations offer comprehensive health services to subscribers, with an emphasis on prevention as well as treatment. Most HMOs have an open enrollment period, usually once a year, when persons may apply for enrollment without medical examination. Some companies have group arrangements with a local HMO, which is an advantage since all employees may enter at standard rates and usually without exclusion by reason of any preexistent condition.

Is group insurance through an association available for a person with epilepsy?

Many organizations and large companies offer group health or life insurance to members, provided a specified number of members take out this insurance. The person with epilepsy should by all means apply for group insurance, for even though the insurance company may ask each applicant to have a physical examination, the insurance premiums are much lower through group plans. Moreover, the person with epilepsy is usually not singled out for higher premiums because of the condition. The person with epilepsy may obtain coverage through a group whereas he might not be given life or health insurance through an individual plan. Most organizations have a probationary period before the new employee or member is eligible to qualify.

It is usually desirable for the person to convert any existing group insurance coverage to an individual policy immediately if there is a change in employment or membership in the association sponsoring the group insurance.

Can the person with epilepsy obtain automobile insurance?

Automobile insurance provides liability, collision, and comprehensive coverage, and medical benefits in case of an accident. Although the conditions under which persons with epilepsy may obtain automobile insurance vary widely from state to state, persons whose seizures are under control are often eligible to obtain such insurance, though usually on an "assigned risk" basis.

Insurance companies generally do not consider a person with epilepsy eligible under a regular auto policy, because of the greater risk involved, and require the agent to apply under the assigned risk plan. Assigned risk coverage is for a specific term (normally three years), after which time the applicant must again apply through his agent for another assigned risk plan if he is not able to obtain standard coverage. A person deemed eligible for assigned risk coverage cannot choose the company that will provide the insurance. As a result, there are wide variations in the rates. Assigned risk plan rates are generally 25 to 50 percent higher than regular insurance rates and may not include collision and comprehensive coverage. The amount of coverage under the assigned risk plan is customarily the minimum limit required by the automobile financial responsibility law in the particular state.

Currently, assigned risk auto insurance is available in all states, but a few states exclude persons with epilepsy from participation. Consequently, in these states a person with epilepsy is allowed to drive but is unable to obtain accident insurance.

Don't the automobile insurance companies actually encourage the person with epilepsy to misrepresent his condition?

To some extent this is true. Disproportionately high auto insurance rates are imposed on persons with epilepsy by insurance companies, so that most persons with a history of seizures, even though they have been controlled for years, must still pay double the standard premium. Consequently, many people are tempted to conceal a history of epilepsy.

What about Social Security disability insurance?

The Social Security Act under Title II, Social Security Disability Insurance, provides disability insurance for employed persons and their families. The program provides cash benefits to workers who become disabled, including those who develop epilepsy, and to dependent disabled adults who develop epilepsy before the age of eighteen.

A parent who must provide extensive care for a disabled dependent adult may also receive cash payments. These payments are made from employer and employee contributions to the Old Age, Survivors, and Disability Insurance (OASDI). If the worker paid into OASDI for a sufficient time and became disabled or died or has a disabled adult relative unable to provide for himself, that person or spouse will probably be eligible for benefits.

The payments, since July 1980, range from approximately $139.50 to $647 per month, depending upon the earnings prior to the disabling condition; family benefits go as high as $970.50. Amounts are adjusted to reflect changes in the cost of living. The disabled dependent receives monthly benefits that range depending on whether the parent has retired or is disabled, or has died. Disabled dependents also become eligible for Medicare health insurance after two years of disability benefits.

Is a person with epilepsy eligible for disability income protection insurance?

In addition to disability coverage through Social Security and Worker's Compensation, and compulsory disability benefits available in a few states (California, New Jersey, New York, Rhode Island), there are some group income protection policies for persons who become disabled while employed. These policies are usually available through relatively large companies. If this protection is desired, it is to the advantage of the person with epilepsy to apply for the group policy, since individual disability income insurance coverage is far more difficult to obtain.

Are any benefits available under Medicare?

Medicare is a federal health insurance program set up through the Social Security Act to help people sixty-five years old and above with the cost of health care. Coverage is available as well to disabled people under the age of sixty-five who have been entitled to Social Security benefits for at least 24 consecutive months. If you have been receiving these benefits for this length of time, you will automatically get Medicare hospital insurance and will receive information about it several months before the coverage becomes effective. The insurance covers hospital inpatient care, medication and other services supplied during the hospitalization, and some part-time services from a home health agency. It does not cover doctors' fees or drugs prescribed outside of the hospital setting. Moreover, if you qualify for the hospital insurance, you also automatically get Medicare medical insurance, which you may choose not to take since it does require the payment of a monthly premium. The medical insurance will cover doctors' fees and other services but not prescription drugs.

There are many aspects to Medicare coverage under both the hospital and the medical insurance programs. For further information, call or write to your local Social Security office.

Can the person with epilepsy expect as long a life as the one without it?

With improved care and treatment, a larger number of persons with epilepsy has attained better seizure control than that of even just a few years ago. Presumably, this would lead to an increase in the life span.

The literature dealing with the life expectancy of those with epilepsy is generally outdated and complicated by problems of determining whether epilepsy was the direct cause of death, or a contributing cause, or was unrelated to the death. A few studies have compared the death rates of people with epilepsy to those without epilepsy. Henriksen (1970) gives some preliminary data on a continuing long-term study that shows the average age of death of the control group is 51.9 years and that of the epilepsy group is 45.3 years, with a difference of 6.6 years. This information is based on the early deaths in the two groups and may change since the majority of both groups are still alive. Several researchers reviewed data from insurance companies and concluded that their results show an overall mortality for policyholders with epilepsy of two to three times greater than the mortality rate expected for a comparable group of policyholders without epilepsy. Again, it must be noted that because a person identified as having epilepsy dies it does not mean that epilepsy was the cause. In fact, the Metropolitan Life Insurance Company considers epilepsy to be only a minor cause of death, and the number of persons who die from it to be lower than that of persons who die from appendectomies.

Most studies show that the mortality rates for persons with epilepsy are related to the person's age. The highest mortality rate is for those under the age of five. The next highest rate is for those over sixty-five, though this of course adds the complications of aging to epilepsy as a cause of death. The third highest mortality is for those between twenty-five and forty-five, with the major causes of death being major seizures, cancer, and accidents.

In general, the average life span of persons with epilepsy seems to be slightly below that of the general population. Those with severe and uncontrolled epilepsy clearly have a higher death rate. Also, the earlier the onset of epilepsy in the life of a person, the higher the mortality rate. Those who acquired the disorder after age thirty are found statistically to have a normal life expectancy.

10

ISSUES

Can a person with epilepsy obtain a license to drive a car?

State licensing statutes generally prohibit the issuance of a license to persons whose driving would be considered a danger to the public safety. The safety provisions apply to persons with physical or mental disabilities (heart disease, chronic alcoholism, etc.) that would make them unsafe drivers. This regulation is applicable to persons with epilepsy as well. Obviously, a person presents a danger to himself, to passengers, and to others if he experiences a seizure while driving an automobile.

The state departments issuing licenses have the responsibility to withhold or withdraw licenses from those persons determined to represent a hazard because of any condition causing lapses of consciousness and control of behavior. However, it is the practice to permit licensure to those whose condition is determined to have been adequately controlled for a reasonable period of time. Some states have a flexible policy, using the judgment of the administrative officer or a medical advisory board in determining whether a person may be issued a license to drive. The officer or board will assess the specific condition of each person with epilepsy, the primary responsibility being to determine whether the applicant's condition is adequately controlled and further seizure activity unlikely.

Most states require a physician's statement of seizure control. Most states also require a complete medical history and an examination of the driving skills and fitness to operate a motor vehicle in a safe manner.

Some states require specific periods of seizure control for the person to be eligible for a license, and these periods are subject to change. The chart at the end of this chapter shows the present seizure-free period (with or without medication) required in each state by statute or regulation, as well as whether periodic medical reports are required and if so at what intervals.

England requires a seizure-free period of three years before a license can be issued. Canada has no time period and evaluates each case separately by a medical review board, which is strict in approving licenses.

Some states require physicians to report all cases of epilepsy or other disorders involving lapses of consciousness to a central agency such as the department of health or the department of motor vehicles. At present, the states mandating such reporting are California, Connecticut, Delaware, Illinois, Indiana, Montana, Nevada, New Jersey, and Oregon. Indeed, without such reporting, many officials issuing licenses would be unable to determine whether a person actually had epilepsy. The incidence of those who do not mention their condition to the licensing official is evidently very high, though statistics are not available here.

The state motor vehicle department may suspend or revoke the driver's license of a person who is reported as having seizures not previously known at the time of licensure. An examining officer will review the circumstances and determine the degree of danger to public safety. A probationary license may be issued. Licenses may also be issued with whatever restrictions are determined appropriate to ensure the safe operation of a motor vehicle. In some states, limited driving privileges permit the person with epilepsy to use a car for essential driving under specified conditions.

Some states require periodic medical reports as a condition of maintaining the driver's license. Most states provide for an indefinite suspension of the license when a person with epilepsy is involved in an accident shown to be related to the condition.

Persons denied a driver's license by the state agency may generally obtain a judicial review of the decision, so, as a rule of thumb, we could say that a person with epilepsy *can* get a driver's license provided that he can establish that the condition is under control.

Persons with epilepsy have been shown to have increased traffic violations and higher accident rates when compared with other drivers. Not all of these are due directly to seizures since other factors contribute to the accident rate, such as sedative side effects of some anticonvulsants.

The British Epilepsy Association's Medical Advisory Committee has made the following recommendations for drivers known to have epilepsy:

1. Avoid driving when tired or for long hours at a time.
2. Avoid driving for long periods without food or sleep.
3. Remember to take the prescribed anticonvulsants regularly when driving, just as when not driving.
4. When one is driving, a petit mal attack is often as danger-ous as grand mal, and one whose petit mal attacks are not controlled should not drive.
5. Anyone taking anticonvulsants should *never* have alcohol in any form when driving, regardless of the quantity.

Can anything be done to help the person with epilepsy get transportation when he is unable to obtain a driver's license?

Transportation is a major problem for those persons unable to obtain a driver's license. Common, everyday journeys such as going shopping or to work or to recreational events, taken for granted by most persons, become extremely difficult when one is unable to drive. Public transportation is frequently crowded, unreliable, or nonexistent. Persons with epilepsy may be reluctant to use a bus or subway for fear of having a seizure. Use of private transportation such as a taxi is too expensive for routine travel. Reliance on relatives or friends and walking often become the major modes of transportation.

The problem has yet to be resolved, though a few alternatives are being developed. Most significant is the Dial-A-Ride mini-bus service, which was designed for this purpose. The Dial-A-Ride programs provide reasonable door-to-door service for shopping, medical appointments, etc., and have been found to operate very successfully in urban areas.

Is a person liable to others for injury inflicted during a seizure?

The question of liability is a complicated one and cannot be answered here in a truly comprehensive way. Liability in regard to a traffic accident may depend upon specific state laws for licensing of drivers; an accident caused by or occurring to a person with epilepsy while on the job may present other aspects of liability. Basically, a person with epilepsy has a responsibility to keep seizure activity reasonably controlled or warn others if it is not. Like diabetics or stroke or heart-disease victims, persons with epilepsy should make reasonable efforts neither to imperil others nor to put themselves in situations of undue risk. In general, we recommend that you consult a lawyer regarding any specific problem.

One thing might be stressed, however: the incidence of persons inflicting bodily harm on others during a seizure is very small. The psychological harm done to those with epilepsy by stigmatizing them as "potentially dangerous" is great. Efforts are being made to remove such social and discriminatory burdens from those who have seizure disorders.

What about hunting or fishing licenses for those with epilepsy?

As in the case of driving licenses, the rules vary from state to state, depending upon the proof of control of seizures and the period of seizure-free activity. The reason for the caution in issuing fishing licenses is the danger of drowning or injury during a seizure. Some states provide free fishing permits and licenses to developmentally disabled persons (including those with epilepsy). To be eligible for these, the person must be a resident of a state institution or family care home, or must provide proof of disability. The permits are generally obtained through application to the state fish and game department. Permits may be issued for fishing independently or under supervision. One may check with the nearest forestry or fish and game department for details.

Hunting licenses, understandably, are more difficult to obtain and usually require a statement from the treating physician.

Should a person with epilepsy carry medical identification?

The decision to wear an identification bracelet or carry an identification medical card indicating that one has a convulsive disorder is up to each individual. There is no legislation requiring that it be done. However, there are certain circumstances in which it would be highly advisable: for children with uncontrolled seizures; for adults with psychomotor epilepsy where periods of confusion may be part of the attack; with generalized tonic-clonic seizures, where the person may require heavy medication that results in drowsiness or difficulty in locomotion. The identification is useful for an emergency room staff, especially during the night or weekends when access to the medical records may not be easy. Also, persons with epilepsy have been arrested by police because of unusual behavior assumed to be caused by alcoholic intoxication.

Several types of identification are in common use. One is an identification plate which may be worn as a bracelet or necklace. These may be obtained through the Medic Alert International Foundation, which supplies the bracelet containing the Medic Alert emblem on one side and the type of disorder on the other. The foundation also records the personal medical history and maintains a twenty-four-hour service for physicians to obtain the pertinent information by phone in case of emergency. This is actually a worldwide answering service. There are several types and styles of emblems for both men and women, all of which would be considered attractive. To order a Medic Alert plate, write to Medic Alert Foundation, P.O. Box 1009, Turlock, California 95380. The lifetime membership fee is $10.

A similar medical identification badge designed to be worn on any watchband is IDenti-Clip. It is inexpensive, designed to hold six lines of emergency medical information, and may be obtained with or without the medical symbol. To order, write to IDenti-Clip, P.O. Box 123, Beaverton, Oregon 97005.

An identification card can be carried in the wallet or purse. The card has the advantage of containing more information and being less conspicuous than a bracelet. However, the card may not be noticed. It is advisable to include the following information on the identification card: your name, address, and phone number; your physician's name, address and phone number; the name of and dosage of medication; and any other significant medical information. Emergency identification cards may be obtained from the American Medical Association, 535 North Dearborn Street, Chicago, Illinois 60610.

We recommend that a person with epilepsy and especially those with a history of "surprise" seizures have both the bracelet and the wallet or purse card.

Can personal identification cards be obtained?

Most states now provide legal identification cards for persons who are not able to obtain a driver's license. The card is valuable for business purposes and for verification of age. Generally, the personal identification cards are issued by the state department of motor vehicles to those who do not have or are not eligible for a license to drive. The cards contain information such as legal name, address, birth date, physical characteristics and/or photograph, and signature. They do not indicate a handicap. These cards should not be confused with medical identification cards, which provide pertinent information regarding the handicap.

Persons age sixteen and over may obtain a personal identification card by applying to the department of motor vehicles in the state of residence.

Can a person with epilepsy marry without a special examination?

Yes. In the past, several states maintained archaic laws preventing marriage of a person with epilepsy, but since 1969 *all* states allow marriage without consideration of the condition of epilepsy.

Is sterilization ever indicated for one with epilepsy?

There should be no involuntary sterilization on the basis of epilepsy. However, as of 1976 several states (Arizona, Delaware, Oklahoma, South Carolina, and Utah) still authorized the involuntary sterilization of institutionalized persons with epilepsy under certain conditions. Generally, these laws require specific reasons for the action and additional, mental handicaps besides the condition of epilepsy.

Women with epilepsy may voluntarily choose sterilization for reasons of health or as a means of birth control.

Can a child with epilepsy be adopted?

Persons may knowingly adopt children with handicaps of all types. However, two states (Arkansas and Missouri) allow annulment of the adoption if the epilepsy is discovered within five years after adoption, provided the adoptive parents were unaware of the seizure condition at the time they acquired the child.

Can a person with epilepsy enlist in the armed forces?

In general, all branches of the military consider epilepsy as grounds for ineligibility. If the applicant had febrile seizures before the age of five with no recurrence after that age, the condition would not exclude him from service. The regulation regarding medical unfitness for enlistment specifies paroxysmal convulsive disorders that include a "disturbance of consciousness, all forms of psychomotor or temporal lobe epilepsy or history thereof, except for seizures associated with toxic states or fever during childhood up to age five." When one enlists in the military and keeps the condition secret, he is subject to discharge without disability compensation when the condition is discovered.

If the person with epilepsy has a special skill that is described as "urgently needed" (for instance, if he is a dentist or lawyer or doctor), he may be admitted for "limited service," provided the seizures are controlled and the person does not require regular clinical or laboratory work-ups.

If one already in the military develops epilepsy, is he discharged? Is he entitled to disability compensation benefits?

If the person is accepted into the military and has a seizure within four months after enlistment, he is generally subject to a medical evaluation, a review by the medical board and the disability review board, and is usually given an "administrative separation" (honorable). However, if the disorder appears *after* the four-month period, he *may* remain on a volunteer basis, provided the seizures are controlled by nontoxic drugs. The person is usually given a limited assignment in which a sudden loss of consciousness would not endanger himself or others. Each case, however, is evaluated separately, with the decision based upon the medical condition and the ability of the person to perform the duties assigned. The four-month period is considered a primary basis for determining whether the person entered the service with the disorder, or whether it was incurred or aggravated while on the job and, therefore, is "service connected." An accident, such as a blow to the head that happened while one was on duty during the first four months, would be considered service connected.

If after the four-month period the person develops a seizure disorder that requires discharge from the service, the disorder is considered service related, and the person is entitled to disability compensation benefits.

Some branches (the Air Force and the Navy being the most stringent) consider that a member who needs prolonged and regular treatment with anticonvulsants may not be eligible for duty restrictions and would be discharged. However, if the person has served sixteen years or more, he may be granted a permanent limited assignment, provided there are no other complicating factors involved.

Are Supplemental Security Income benefits affected when one's condition is so severe as to require institutionalization?

Though SSI benefits are available to those persons with epilepsy who have very low personal incomes, benefits are decreased by one third if the person is placed in a group home. If, however, the person must be placed in a public hospital setting, the SSI payments automatically end. The EFA feels, and the authors of this book certainly agree, that this system virtually makes institutionalization a permanent way of life, leaving the individual little alternative but to remain institutionalized.

The Nationwide Plan includes provisions to remedy this situation that are listed in the Epilogue (see Living Arrangements: Community Housing).

I understand there are some inequities in financial assistance to those with epilepsy. Is this true?

Unfortunately, it *is* true that there are several inequities. For one, the beneficiary of Social Security disability insurance must receive disability benefits for 24 months before obtaining Medicare coverage. Furthermore, since Medicare coverage for anticonvulsants is available only on an inpatient basis, many persons with epilepsy have a greater incentive for hospitalization than is normally necessary. In addition, under Medicaid, anticonvulsants are an optional service, covered in some states and not in others.

Another inequity lies in the fact that if seizures are controlled through treatment and medication, the person no longer qualifies as "disabled" under either disability insurance or SSI, yet no allowance is made as to whether the person is employed or has an income to take the place of the lost benefits. Furthermore, those persons who have controlled seizures are no longer classified as "severely disabled" and thus no longer qualify for priority in vocational rehabilitation services, making their difficulties in obtaining jobs even more pronounced. Though Medicare and Medicaid may cover the cost of anticonvulsants when one has seizures, this coverage is lost when the seizures are under control. This creates a sad cycle of reoccurrence of seizures when there is no money for medication to control them.

Recently, several changes have been made in the Social Security disability program to assist those with epilepsy who return to work. Medicare coverage is extended for a 36-month period, even if the benefits have been suspended because earnings have gone over the eligibility limit. Also, the first two years of employment are considered a trial work period. During the second half of this period, the person does not receive benefits if the earnings are more than the allowed amount, but the eligibility remains if the person should be forced to return to disability allowances. Additionally, work-related expenses, such as the cost of anticonvulsants needed to make employment possible, are no longer counted as part of the earnings that would cause loss of benefits.

The Commission for the Control of Epilepsy and Its Consequences has made many strong recommendations for the Nationwide Plan to resolve the financial inequities (see the Epilogue under Independence and Equality: Financial Assistance).

Is one's employment affected by epilepsy?

Authorities have written that the two problems second only to the seizures themselves are social adjustment and employment. However, depending on the nature and severity of the seizures and the degree of control, these two problems can be partially solved. A recent study in England showed that 80 percent of persons of normal intelligence with epilepsy were satisfactorily employed. They found the prognosis for complete social adjustment and employment was somewhat worse for those with temporal lobe epilepsy and for those with frequent seizures beginning in childhood. The major causes of unemployment reported in this study were (1) impairment of intellectual functioning and (2) personality difficulties, which may or may not be associated with epilepsy.

A 1973 survey of employment possibilities made by the Epilepsy Foundation of America was not as encouraging as the British study. The EFA found that 46 percent of persons with epilepsy had been refused employment because of the disorder, 30 percent had been dismissed from their jobs because of seizures, and 45 percent stated that their choice of occupation had been influenced by their having epilepsy.

The attitudes of employers in the survey were significant in terms of acceptance of seizures. Forty percent of the persons with epilepsy reported that their employers reacted in a positive and supportive manner to seizures at work. Twenty-five percent reported, however, that seizures were directly responsible for their dismissal, early retirement, or lack of advancement. The respondents in the EFA survey reported that nearly half of their co-workers reacted realistically to a seizure, while approximately one third reacted with fear, fright, or panic.

The unemployment rate among those with epilepsy is needlessly high and results in a tragic loss of talent and productivity. At present, estimates of the overall unemployment rate for those known to have epilepsy and not living in any institution come to 25 percent. This figure runs much higher during periods of general unemployment.

One key factor is unemployment is the attitude and emotional well-being of the person with epilepsy. Individuals without jobs tend to be discouraged and lose confidence in themselves. With such feelings interest in taking the medication declines, and consequently more seizures occur. In turn, there is then less opportunity for employment; and despondency and withdrawal become more severe; interest in searching for a job or acquiring new skills is inhibited; and the cycle of unemployment continues.

The feelings and attitudes a person has toward his epilepsy are critical in obtaining and holding a job. Many employment problems could be prevented with proper vocational counseling and a focus on the person involved in the employment process. At the same time, employers and the general public need enlightenment. Unfortunately, the person with epilepsy *is* often penalized by the disorder.

What are the problems in employment?

Discrimination in employment is still a major concern although a number of positive changes have occurred in recent years. Federal legislation under Sections 501, 503, and 504 of the Rehabilitation Act of 1973 provides guidelines to be followed by those employers who have federal contracts or agencies with federally funded programs. Section 501 prohibits discrimination on the basis of a handicap for all federal employees except the military and requires each federal agency to take steps to hire and promote qualified handicapped persons. Section 503 prevents discriminatory employment practices and provides affirmative action guides for employment of handicapped in private companies that obtain federal contracts. Section 504 requires employers with federal grants and programs to refrain from employment discrimination and to make reasonable modifications in job functions to accommodate handicapped persons. Complaints regarding these areas may be registered with any federal office of civil rights.

Some employers are still reluctant to hire persons with epilepsy and occasionally reject an applicant because of a history of epilepsy not reported on the job application. Thus a person with controlled seizures may be prevented from obtaining employment. Other employers believe that their insurance rates will go up if they hire someone with epilepsy. However, workers' compensation rates are determined by the industrial classes of jobs, conditions at the worksite, and the total accident history of the employer. The hiring of someone with epilepsy who can safely perform the job will not cause an increase in workers' compensation premiums.

All public and private employers covered by the Rehabilitation Act of 1973 (Sections 501, 502, 503) must comply with regulations that prohibit illegal employment discrimination in hiring, promotion, and termination, and are required to make reasonable modifications of the job to allow person with handicapping conditions, such as epilepsy, to perform the job. Most states also have adopted laws preventing employment discrimination against the handicapped.* State laws vary as to who is protected and what obligations are placed on employers. State statutes apply to many employers not covered by the federal Rehabilitation Act. Thus, most workers now have some protection against employment discrimination.

Employers can make all types of personnel decisions regarding their employees except illegally discriminatory ones. For a personnel decision to be "illegally discriminatory," it must have the effect of discriminating against a member of a "protected class," such as a handicapped individual, solely on tbe basis of the handicap and

---

*Forty states have such laws; the ten that do not are Alabama, Arizona, Arkansas, Delaware, Mississippi, North Dakota, Oklahoma, South Carolina, South Dakota, and Wyoming.

without any relation to the real requirements of the job. (Other "protected classes" are race, national origin, age, sex, and religion.)

Those necessary elements of a job that are related to performance are known as "bona fide occupational qualifications" (BFOQ). These have been established by court rulings addressing challenges brought by unsuccessful candidates for jobs. For example, employment as an airline pilot could be denied to an otherwise qualified person with uncontrolled seizures, for here the employer would be able to show that remaining conscious and alert (a BFOQ for this position) is necessary to pilot the plane, and no reasonable alteration of this requirement could be made without significant hazards. Anyone not having a BFOQ for a job need not be hired.

Employers must, however, make reasonable accommodations at the worksite to allow handicapped persons to perform jobs. A "reasonable accommodation" may involve adaptation of the work environment, equipment, or duties to allow the handicapped person to perform in a safe manner. Accommodations are considered reasonable if they do not impose undue financial hardship on the employer. For example, accommodation for persons with epilepsy might include a readjustment of scheduling or a modification of the job duties.

The Rehabilitation Act limits and defines the preemployment questions that employers may ask and removes from job applications questions about epilepsy. While an employer cannot, then, specifically ask about epilepsy, he may ask applicants if they can safely perform job-related functions. The job applicant is not obligated to inform the employer about the condition or history of epilepsy if that condition presents no hazard. A preemployment medical examination may be done if it is required of all employees and only after a conditional offer of employment has been made. At the present time, a person with epilepsy that is not fully controlled should discuss the implications of the condition with the prospective employer, and they should together work out an acceptable accommodation on the job. Important factors include a careful analysis of the working conditions, the seizure type and frequency, medication taken and its side effects, and a plan to adapt the job specifications to take these factors into account. It is reasonable for the employer to expect an employee to perform successfully the job for which he or she is hired. Persons who are currently seizure-free and for whom recurrence is unlikely, as well as those who had epilepsy in childhood only, need not inform the employer in any event. Recent court cases have required the employment of a policeman and a respiratory therapist who were previously denied employment because of a history of epilepsy.

It should be noted that the entire field of employment discrimination regarding the handicapped is novel and will undoubtedly undergo additional refinement through new court decisions and clarification of regulations. Many important issues are still unsettled, such as what constitutes an acceptable degree of risk and how much accommodation is reasonable.

If you find that an employer is reluctant to hire you, provide him or her with some literature on epilepsy; discuss obligations toward your condition; and suggest some possible accommodations. Additionally, have your vocational rehabilitation counselor or physician contact the company on your behalf. Remember that the law merely makes epilepsy a neutral factor in hiring. It does not afford an undue advantage to the handicapped, and it protects the handicapped worker only in that the handicap does not prevent him or her from performing the essential functions of a job on a competitive basis with other employees.

Are plans under way to improve the job placement opportunities for persons with epilepsy?

The Commission for the Control of Epilepsy and Its Consequences has made many strong recommendations in this area, which are reported in greater depth in the Epilogue.

The actual job placement for persons with epilepsy has, in truth, suffered greatly in the past. The commission cites a number of reasons for difficulty in this area, most of which are common knowledge, and which are based largely on the reluctance of employers to hire anyone who may represent a potential "problem." Many company physicians have been known to recommend against hiring, purely on the basis of epilepsy, without giving any individual considerations. Besides the specific recommendations listed in the Epilogue, however, a few notable programs are in effect that have been found successful:

PWI. Projects With Industry is a federally funded program that uses company coordinators to place handicapped persons in industry.

TAPS. Training and Placement Service, run by the Epilepsy Foundation of America and funded by contract with the Department of Labor, has been successful in training and placing persons with epilepsy in industry.

Employment Office. Job placement is also available through the public employment offices of the Department of Labor. Local offices are available in most communities to serve those seeking employment. Each office has a designated person to assist the handicapped.

The commission has recommended to the Department of Labor that handicapped persons, including those with epilepsy, be designated as a "special group," under the CETA regulations. The specific recommendations of the commission are listed in the Epilogue under Job Placement. If carried out, they should resolve many of the problems of job placement of those with epilepsy in the near future.

What is the Commission for the Control of Epilepsy and its consequences?

The commission was established on July 29, 1975, under Public Law 94-63, and was composed of nine members with life service in and prestigious contribution to the field of epilepsy. The commission was given four major mandates:

1. To survey the medical and social management of epilepsy
2. To make recommendations regarding research, prevention, identification, and rehabilitation
3. To develop a comprehensive Nationwide Plan for the control of epilepsy and its consequences
4. To make recommendations for the prevention and control of epilepsy and its consequences

On August 1, 1977, the commission presented its completed report to the Congress and the President. The commission ended its mammoth work with three strong convictions:

1. The incidence of epilepsy can be reduced by a series of relatively inexpensive preventive measures if the public can be convinced of the necessity of these measures.
2. The quality of care can be substantially improved for a large percentage of those with epilepsy by continuing investment in basic and clinical research, and by more rapid and efficient transfer of technology.
3. Through comprehensive educational programs in both the public and private sectors, necessary services can be made more responsive to the unique problems of epilepsy and can be more accessible financially and geographically to those who need them, thus reducing the medical and social consequences of epilepsy.

The commission is to be congratulated on completing such an undertaking in only two years, and it is now our hope that their recommendations will be followed as soon as possible.

What is the so-called Nationwide Plan for Action on Epilepsy? Is it as far-reaching as I have heard?

The commission (discussed in the previous question) had as its purpose the establishment of a Nationwide Plan, which is in truth more far-reaching than many of its proponents had hoped. This comprehensive Plan seeks to unify the various programs in the several states into one national plan for combating epilepsy and its consequences. (The commission noted that in 41 of the 50 states there "appeared to be no focal point for program development to meet the unique needs of persons with epilepsy.")

The overall purpose of the Plan was to "enable the people of the United States and its Territories to achieve effective prevention and control of epilepsy, and to reduce the negative impact of the consequences of epilepsy both for individuals and their families and for the nation as a whole." The commission developed two specific goals on which to base its recommendations for the Plan:

1. To reduce substantially the number of people who suffer from epilepsy by discovering and applying effective methods for the prevention of the various forms of epilepsy.
2. To control seizures and to ameliorate their impact so that affected individuals may attain, as much as possible
   a. good health,
   b. living in the least restricted environment,
   c. satisfying work at an appropriate level of skill,
   d. financial security, and
   e. social adjustment.

The commission's four-volume report was published in August of 1977. Volume I presents the Nationwide Plan itself, which includes more than 400 recommendations in the major areas that affect persons with epilepsy. (These recommendations are summarized in the Epilogue.) Volume II deals primarily with the research proposals, the basic material on which the recommendations are based. Volume III studies the various federal, state, and voluntary resources. Volume IV deals largely with the economics involved.

The major objectives of the Plan are as follows (condensed from *Plan for Nationwide Action on Epilepsy,* Volume I):

1. To reduce by 1982 the overall incidence of epilepsy by 15 percent and the frequency of seizures by 25 percent
2. To achieve by 1980 greater understanding of the causes of epilepsy and to develop improved techniques for prevention, diagnosis, treatment, and control through research
3. To assure by 1980 that every individual with epilepsy will receive adequate medical services
4. To ease by 1980 the social adjustment and mental health of all individuals with epilepsy and their families in order to optimize their total life functioning
5. To provide improved education, training, and employment opportunities

6. To provide by 1980 a substantial increase in the possibilities for independent living and equality as guaranteed by law

7. To assure by 1980 a continuum of services and a variety of living arrangements for each individual with epilepsy

8. To achieve by 1982 a 25 percent increase in compliance with medical regimens, a 25 percent reduction in the number of untreated cases of epilepsy, a 25 percent reduction in the occurrence of status epilepticus, and a 25 percent reduction in the frequency of seizures

9. To develop by 1982 a Comprehensive Epilepsy Services Network

As mentioned, the specific recommendations under the nine major objectives listed above are spelled out in the Epilogue. The importance of the recommendations cannot be overemphasized. As Dr. Richard Masland, Executive Director of the commission, writes, "It is a new day for handicapped people in the United States." James Autry, President of the Epilepsy Foundation of America, carried it even farther. He wrote, "We have a national plan for action on epilepsy. Now, we must make sure that the plan becomes a reality."

STATE REQUIREMENTS FOR ELIGIBILITY FOR DRIVER'S LICENSE

STATE	SEIZURE-FREE PERIOD	PERIODIC MEDICAL REPORTS REQUIRED
Alabama	1 year (administrative policy)	Every year from physician for 10 years from date of last seizure.
Alaska	1 year with statement from physician.	At renewal every 5 years with statement from physician.

STATE	SEIZURE-FREE PERIOD	PERIODIC MEDICAL REPORTS REQUIRED
Arizona	1 year on medication, 2 years off medication; both with report from Arizona physician.	3-year renewal with letter from Arizona physician.
Arkansas	1 year	None
California	None. Medical clearance required that seizures are under control. Individual consideration given for type of restricted license.	At intervals, determined by Department of Motor Vehicles (usually every 6 or 12 months) until seizure-free for 3 years.
Colorado	1 year	As deemed necessary by physician or license examiner.
Connecticut	2 years	According to attending physician's recommendation.
Delaware	None. Medical release to drive must be obtained from 2 physicians.	Yearly, until medical certification of cure.
District of Columbia	1 year	Yearly
Florida	1 year with medical statement; 2 years without medical statement.	Yearly until seizure-free for 2 years.
Georgia	1-year guideline	None
Hawaii	None. Medical release to drive.	None
Idaho	6 months to 2 years	None
Illinois	None. Medical release to drive.	As often as physician or Medical Review Board deems necessary.
Indiana	1 year	None

STATE	SEIZURE-FREE PERIOD	PERIODIC MEDICAL REPORTS REQUIRED
Iowa	6 months with report from physician.	Every 2 years with letter from physician.
Kansas	1 year	Each time license renewed.
Kentucky	3 months	As deemed necessary by medical examiner.
Louisiana	1 year with report from physician.	Renewal every 2 years with report from physician.
Maine	1 year	As deemed necessary by Medical Coordinator.
Maryland	1 year	May be required by Medical Advisory Board.
Massachusetts	18 months	On individual basis, from every 6 months to every year. Report must be from a neurologist.
Michigan	1 year with report from physician.	Renewal every 4 years with statement from physician.
Minnesota	1 year	Yearly until seizure-free for 2 to 3 years, then every 2 to 4 years.
Mississippi	1 year	None
Missouri	None. Medical release to drive.	None
Montana	None. Must be seizure-free; records sent by recognized doctor to Highway Patrol, which decides if person may take driver's test.	None
Nebraska	1 year with report from physician.	None. Renewal with statement from physician.

STATE	SEIZURE-FREE PERIOD	PERIODIC MEDICAL REPORTS REQUIRED
Nevada	1 year with or without medication; report from physician.	[Unknown]
New Hampshire	1 year. Letter from doctor required.	As deemed necessary
New Jersey	1 year	Every 6 months until seizure-free for 3–5 years.
New Mexico	2 years	None
New York	1 year	At 4-year intervals.
North Carolina	1 year	Voluntary self-report yearly.
North Dakota	Restricted license; 6 months with medical certification.	Yearly until seizure-free for 5 years.
Ohio	None. Medical release to drive.	Every 6 months for 1 year; then annually until seizure-free for 4 years.
Oklahoma	1 year	At renewal; 1 or 2 years.
Oregon	Variable; based upon medical recommendation; 3 to 12 months for patients with recurrent seizures after treatment.	Yearly until seizure-free for 2 years.
Pennsylvania	1 year	None
Rhode Island	None. Medical approval by Registry of Motor Vehicles, Medical Advisory Board.	None
South Carolina	1 year	Every 6 months until seizure-free for 3 years.

STATE	SEIZURE-FREE PERIOD	PERIODIC MEDICAL REPORTS REQUIRED
South Dakota	18 months with report from physician.	None
Tennessee	2 years; with special approval of Medical Review Board and physician, person may be allowed to take licensing exam after being seizure-free for 1 year.	None
Texas	Individual consideration by Medical Advisory Board; guideline is seizure-free for 1 year.	As deemed necessary by Medical Advisory Board.
Utah	3 months with area and daytime driving limitation; 6 months unrestricted.	Every 6 months until seizure-free for 5 years.
Vermont	24 months; Commissioner may grant conditional license after person is seizure-free for 6 months with good prognosis from medical consultant.	Every 6 months until seizure-free for 2 years.
Virginia	1 year	Every 1 or 2 years depending upon physician's recommendation.
Washington	6 months seizure-free with medical report.	Medical examinations may be imposed in 6-month, 12-month, or 24-month cycles.
West Virginia	1 year	Every year for 2 years, then frequency of medical reports relaxed somewhat, depending upon individual.

STATE	SEIZURE-FREE PERIOD	PERIODIC MEDICAL REPORTS REQUIRED
Wisconsin	6 months	Every 6 months for 2 years; then yearly until seizure-free for 5 years.
Wyoming	1 year	Yearly
Puerto Rico	None. Medical release to drive.	At 4-year renewal.

11

EPILOGUE

What activities are currently under way that might give those with epilepsy greater hope for the future?

When one considers that more than two million Americans have epilepsy, making it second in number only to mental retardation, it seems strange that research and public interest were so long in coming. It is especially remarkable since the epilepsy movement in our country began in the 1890s! Several agencies, however, have rapidly developed research projects and are disseminating information to the public to the extent that old prejudices and stereotypes are gradually becoming a thing of the past. Most notable in this effort have been the Epilepsy Foundation of America and the National Institute of Neurological and Communicative Disorders and Stroke (part of the Department of Health and Human Services), though they have had far from an easy road.

There have been some legislative landmarks, beginning in 1945, when epilepsy finally came to the attention of Congress. In testimony before the Subcommittee on Aid to the Physically Handicapped, Dr. William Lennox, one of our strongest advocates, said in part, ". . . of all the handicaps which you and your committees are studying, epilepsy without doubt is the least understood by both the medical and general public, and is the most neglected." He then proposed funds for a national institute for neuropsychiatric research (including epilepsy), a federal grant-in-aid program, and centers for diagnosis, training, and treatment. In 1949, Dr. Lennox again appeared in testimony on behalf of the Epilepsy Act, with the result that in 1950 the United States established the National Institute of Neurological Diseases and Blindness. Eighteen years later, this agency narrowed in on Dr. Lennox's target by becoming the National Institute for Neurological and Communicative Disorders and Stroke.

Little happened until 1963, when epilepsy was finally considered as needing a nationally coordinated effort as a separate entity, and the first Secretary's Meeting (of the Department of Health, Education, and Welfare) on epilepsy was held. The Developmental Disabilities Services and Facilities Construction Amendments of 1970 (PL 91-517), which allotted funds to serve those with "neurological handicaps originating in childhood," was passed in 1971.

This legislation took place nearly three quarters of a century after the epilepsy movement had begun, but it at least established that developmental disabilities (including epilepsy) warranted research and treatment. This legislation was followed in rapid succession by other acts, giving further hope to the cause.

In 1973, the EFA endorsed and encouraged the concept of a national plan. Later the same year, Senator Peter Dominick (R-Colorado) introduced a Joint Resolution in the Senate favoring the establishment of a commission that would, in turn, develop a national plan. The following March, 1974, Representative Peter D. Kyros (D-Maine) introduced a similar measure in the House. Both measures received strong support and in August of the same year, hearings were conducted. The hearings had the support of the EFA, professionals in the field, and victims of epilepsy. Also in 1974, the proposal for an epilepsy commission and a national plan was added to Senator Edward Kennedy's health legislation proposal, a bill that passed both houses only to be vetoed by President Gerald Ford.

In January 1975, the bill was reintroduced and again vetoed by President Ford, but this time the veto was overridden, and the bill became law.

The commission was finally formed and immediately began making the plans that had been so long delayed. Throughout the following eighteen months, special workshops and regional meetings were held to identify the key issues and to make recommendations. The final result was the mammoth four-volume report, *Plan for Nationwide Action on Epilepsy*.

Volume I of this report was condensed in the EFA publication *The National Spokesman* (vol. X, no. 8, 1977) and is recommended reading for those who desire to pursue the Plan in depth. A modified condensation of the EFA summary of the Nationwide Plan recommendations follows:

RECOMMENDATIONS MADE BY THE COMMISSION FOR THE CONTROL OF EPILEPSY AND ITS CONSEQUENCES

I. Prevention

(This is a major concern of the commission mandated by Congress. *Primary* prevention refers to preventing the occurrence of epilepsy, or preventing subsequent seizures by curing the underlying cause. *Secondary* prevention refers to preventing the effects of epilepsy, either by control of seizures or by ameliorating their effects.)

A. *Maternal and Child Health:*
1. The identification of high-risk mothers (for example, women with epilepsy), and establishment of standards of care for all these mothers
2. Training for physicians on the management of pregnant women with epilepsy, with symposia and continuing education programs
3. Access to expert advice through the epilepsy team concept
4. Access for all pregnant women with epilepsy to a neurologist and to anticonvulsant blood-level monitoring
5. Neurological examinations for high-risk infants
6. A full set of immunizations (if medically advised) as a prerequisite to school attendance

B. *Head Injury Prevention:*
1. Mandatory use of helmets by motorcycle riders
2. Mandatory lap and shoulder belts for auto riders
3. Enforcement of the 55-mph speed limit
4. Prevention of driving under the influence of alcohol
5. Better safety in schools
6. Improved medical techniques for management of head injuries
7. Means leading to earlier identification and control of seizures in children
8. Preparation and distribution of materials on infantile spasms

9. Evaluation of the use of preventive medication after head injury or febrile convulsions
10. More prompt treatment in emergency situations, such as status epilepticus, and distribution of educational materials designed to prevent status epilepticus by close compliance with drug schedules
11. National examinations for physicians, which include questions on anticonvulsants and emergency treatment

C. *Recognition and Screening:*
1. Preparation and dissemination of materials for teachers, parents, school nurses, etc., for early recognition of seizure symptoms
2. Early recognition of the high-risk children, particularly children whose neurological development shows some deficits
3. Early recognition of children with more subtle forms of seizures
4. Investigation of the possibility of a single, comprehensive diagnostic and treatment program for all children
5. Better questionnaires to identify seizures, and materials describing symptoms disseminated for use in mass health screening programs, with a better coordination of screening efforts
6. Encouragement of all states to adopt the special education screening program for three-year-olds (offered by the Education of All Handicapped Children Law)
7. A demonstration project to determine the cost and effectiveness of a supervision program, beginning at birth, for low-income or high-risk children

D. *Permanent Seizure Arrest:*
1. Provision by the proposed epilepsy resource teams of investigation facilities for the detection of brain tumors in patients with severe, intractable epilepsy
2. Planning by Health Systems Agencies for the distribution of CAT scan equipment so that it is available as a diagnostic tool for all persons with epilepsy
3. Study of the impact of vigorous physical activity on seizures
4. A joint effort in connection with voluntary organizations concerned with alcoholism to develop a counseling program regarding the problems of epilepsy and alcohol
5. More study about the efficacy of drugs

II. Research
A. *Clinical Investigation:*
1. More investigation of subgroups (for example, absence

seizures), with continued support of the broad range of clinical studies

2. Research into the phenomenon of sudden death in epilepsy
3. Sleep and respiratory studies
4. A workshop on status epilepticus

B. *Pregnancy:*

1. More study of the relationship between pregnancy and seizures, including a special symposium, a task force to collect data, a center to study biochemical and hormonal factors operating during pregnancy, and a study using the data from the Collaborative Perinatal Project
2. Funded studies to determine the frequency of pregnancy in women with epilepsy, the outcome, and the factors influencing it

C. *Febrile Convulsions:*

1. Research to determine if and when anticonvulsants should be started as a preventive measure in a child who has febrile convulsions
2. Review of the Collaborative Perinatal Study data to determine whether susceptibility to febrile convulsions with complications can be predicted, and whether the use of anticonvulsants is appropriate

D. *Prevention:*

1. Research to develop means for the prevention of epilepsy following an injury to the head
2. A survey of the current medical management of head injuries and their outcome, in selected communities
3. A study (involving both men and women) of those taking anticonvulsants, to determine the effect of the drugs on their newborn infants
4. Research to determine the effects of fetal and neonatal hormones on the development of the central nervous system
5. Research to determine the specific antecedents and predictors of epilepsy
6. Follow-up of the offspring of mothers with epilepsy and children who develop seizures, through the Collaborative Perinatal Project

E. *Allergy and Infectious Diseases:*

1. More study of the relationship of autoimmune mechanisms in epilepsy
2. Establishment of a center to study viral encephalitis and to do brain-tissue analysis
3. Further research to develop a vaccine against meningitis
4. Establishment of a brain-tissue bank to provide tissue for research study

F. *Toxic and Metabolic Factors:*
1. A multidisciplinary study of the management of persons with alcoholism and epilepsy
2. An intensive review of information on the effects of various substances, including lead, so that a surveillance system for environmentally caused neurological disease can be established

G. *Hormonal Factors:*
1. Increased study into the area of susceptibility of persons (especially women and teenagers) to hormonal influence on seizures

H. *Psychological Factors:*
1. Research to examine the emotional problems of persons with epilepsy
2. Establishment of a clinical research unit at the National Institutes of Health to study psychosis in epilepsy and means of preventing it
3. Short-term residential care for persons with epilepsy who also have emotional and psychological problems
4. Establishment of a research center for study of persons with epilepsy and severe behavior problems

I. *Surgical Treatment:*
1. Establishment of a program for the surgical treatment of epilepsy available through the Comprehensive Epilepsy Services Network
2. Research on the pathophysiology of the epileptic discharge
3. Research in brain chemistry to determine how it influences seizures and how it may be manipulated to control seizures

J. *Drug Research:*
1. Continued funding of the NINCDS program for new drug development
2. Continued monitoring of anticonvulsants for their toxic effects, effects on the nervous system, and the problem of drug tolerance
3. Expansion of the NINCDS drug research program, especially on the effects of anticonvulsants on pregnant women, and on the safety of drugs used by children with epilepsy
4. Special consideration for approval of sodium valproate
5. A congressionally appointed commission to study the problems of introducing new drugs in the United States, particularly those with limited market potential

K. *Dissemination of Findings:*
1. Retention of the Epilepsy Abstract Retrieval System for the dissemination of information on epilepsy research, with a

tie-in with the proposed Community Resource Teams and other information systems

L. *Dental Research:*
1. Research as to why phenytoin leads to excessive growth of gum tissue, and how this can be prevented

M. *Related Research:*
1. Review by the National Institute of General Medicine Studies of its program in basic pharmacology to assure that certain drug actions are included in the field of study
2. Extension by the Veterans' Administration of its program of care and research for patients with epilepsy by strengthening its network of epilepsy centers

N. *Health Services Delivery Research:*
1. Designation by the Developmental Disabilities Office of a staff member to be responsible for research on the delivery of services to persons with epilepsy, and development and extension by the Department of Labor of the CETA program, with a similar aim
2. Specific research on rehabilitation of persons with epilepsy, including studies of employer and co-worker attitudes, disclosure problems, and the relative benefits of the various forms of job-entry programs
3. A special project to determine the best ways of working with people with epilepsy, and a study of the best methods of delivering services
4. Dissemination of results of mental health studies on persons with epilepsy throughout the mental health care system
5. Demonstration projects in service delivery and management of children with epilepsy by the proposed epilepsy resource teams
6. A study of adaptive behavior of children in various classroom settings

O. *International Efforts:*
1. A coordinated effort between the International League and the International Bureau to provide a single unifying program to meet universal needs of persons with epilepsy
2. Continuation of the International League's work on a universally applicable classification system
3. Work by the League on test measures to assure that drug test data are universally applicable for evaluation in all countries
4. Fostering and encouragement of international exchange and symposia in epilepsy by the Fogarty International Center at NIH

P. *Budget:*
   1. Increased funds provided by Congress for various research grants, including development of new drugs, training of neurologists, and continued support of the Comprehensive Epilepsy Programs

III. Medical Services
   A. *Minimum Standards:*
      1. Development of minimum standards for essential medical services available for *all* who have epilepsy (this has been done; the commission found that in many instances no minimum standards for care existed)
      2. Periodic monitoring of blood levels, once diagnosis is made and the anticonvulsant prescribed, with not less than three monitorings in the initial diagnostic phase
      3. Availability of emergency facilities for persons with epilepsy on a 24-hour basis
      4. Adoption of minimum care standards by accreditation groups for all with epilepsy
   B. *Provision of Medical Services:*
      1. A study of the distribution and shortage of neurologists in the country and the lack of consultation available to the primary care physicians who treat an estimated 90 percent of patients with epilepsy
      2. Adequate medical services (an estimated 35 percent of urban patients are not receiving adequate services, with the rural patient percentage estimated as far greater)
   C. *Quality Control:*
      1. Continuation of the blood-level monitoring programs under the auspices of the Center for Disease Control when the EFA program comes to an end
      2. Upgrading of the quality of EEG laboratories and interpretation of records
      3. Following of standards established by the American EEG Society and the Joint Commission on the Accreditation of Hospitals
      4. Blue Cross, Blue Shield, and other insurance reimbursement *only* for tests performed at facilities meeting these standards, and Medicare/Medicaid reimbursements only for EEGs in labs meeting the American EEG standards
   D. *Medical Services for Children:*
      1. Development of more effective and coordinated services, with special emphasis on child health
      2. A unique data collection system to report on services and

needs of children by disability, including epilepsy
3. Establishment of minimum standards of care for the federal programs concerned with child health needs, including standards for the treatment of seizure disorders
4. Assurance of community input in the administration of child health programs
5. Plans for coordination of school health services with other local health providers
6. Plans for a federal monitoring of Crippled Children's and Maternal and Child Health programs
7. Encouragement of all states to include epilepsy among conditions eligible for Crippled Children's Services
8. Preparation of technical guidelines on epilepsy to help local agencies improve care
9. Surveying and monitoring by local epilepsy organizations of local agencies for the type and quality of care available to children with epilepsy

IV. Social Adjustment and Mental Health
   A. *General Considerations:*
      1. Wide availability of counseling to persons with epilepsy and their families
      2. A national training program for recreation program personnel in the management of epilepsy
      3. Workshops for local recreation program directors
      4. Efforts by local epilepsy groups to increase the participation of children with epilepsy in their recreation programs
   B. *Severe Problems:*
      1. Coordination of state mental health directors and directors of other appropriate agencies toward a system of mental health services, with specific attention to those with epilepsy
      2. Provision of all essential services outlined in the NIMH guidelines for federally funded Community Mental Health Centers
      3. Availability of medical aid to persons with epilepsy within the state mental health systems, and avoidance of "dumping" of clients between agencies
      4. Data to determine whether medical services are being provided
      5. Training in epilepsy for mental health professionals
      6. Establishment of mechanisms to evaluate and meet the full range of residential needs of persons with epilepsy with mental health problems

7. Monitoring by voluntary organizations of the provision of mental health services in the community

V. Education and Employment
   A. *Preschool Education:*
      1. Education of the handicapped and normal together
      2. Adoption by the states of the option provided in the Education of All Handicapped Children Law and provision of such programs beginning at age three
      3. Cooperation between voluntary epilepsy agencies and Head Start programs in developing manuals and aids related to the problems of children with epilepsy
      4. Federally funded day-care centers and staff required to show understanding of how to handle children with epilepsy
   B. *Elementary Schools:*
      1. A study of classroom placement of children with epilepsy to establish criteria for special placement
      2. Addition of the phrase "handicaps involving seizures" to the regulations of the Education of All Handicapped Children Act, to ensure the inclusion of children with epilepsy
      3. Better education of the school community about epilepsy
      4. Preparation of guides and materials for all teachers on the management of children with epilepsy
      5. Development of methods of assessing and managing learning difficulties in children with epilepsy
      6. Provision for school assessment and correction of perceptual and behavioral difficulties of children with epilepsy, with emphasis on individual attention
      7. Counseling available for the child and his family
      8. Instruction for teachers in how to recognize and deal with gaps in academic achievement
      9. Improved school health services and health education
      10. Cooperation between the schools and health agencies
   C. *Vocational Education:*
      1. Consistency between the eligibility requirements of the Vocational Education Act of 1963 (that 10 percent of each state's basic grant to vocational education should be used for handicapped persons) and the Education of All Handicapped Children Law, with epilepsy clearly included in both
      2. Removal of existing restrictions, and greater clarity in administrative guidelines and evaluation of existing programs

    3. Widening of the provision against discrimination on the basis of sex to include discrimination based on handicapping conditions

D. *Rehabilitation:*

    1. Expansion of rehabilitation services to those with epilepsy

    2. More intensive training for counselors, a revision of the case-closure system, availability of psychological counseling, and follow-up services

    3. Optimal and prompt medical care for seizure control with minimal toxicity, as a priority item for clients with seizures

    4. Addition of an expert on epilepsy to the rehabilitation services staff

    5. Pilot research programs to determine what works best, and how to bring about needed changes

    6. Efforts by state Developmental Disabilities Councils to make sure that state plans address the number and success rate of local vocational rehabilitation programs, detail the training programs available to counselors, and report on the number of institutionalized people with epilepsy who are gainfully employed

    7. Research by voluntary groups to find out to what extent persons with epilepsy are included in the state vocational rehabilitation service policy planning, and to suggest needed changes

E. *Job Placement:*

    1. Designation of persons with epilepsy as a "special group," included in the CETA regulations, and the acquainting of CETA prime sponsors with the special needs of those with epilepsy

    2. Compiling of statistics on employment of the handicapped, including a system of matching job opportunities with the available handicapped persons

    3. Development of more programs like TAPS (the EFA's Training and Placement Service)

    4. Experimenting with a "buddy" system placement method

    5. Involvement by the U.S. Employment Service (USES) of the handicapped in its decisions and programs; USES collection of data on all persons with epilepsy, addition of program specialists for the handicapped, and removal of persons with epilepsy from the "neuropsychiatric" category

    6. A mechanism by which employees shall be informed of their rights under Sections 503 and 504 to prevent discrimination in employment and job practices by agencies and contractors receiving federal funds

7. A check on compliance with affirmative action plans
8. Better cooperation between overlapping agencies
9. Preparation of guidelines to assist industrial physicians regarding the capabilities and employability of persons with epilepsy
10. Urging of unions to provide training for medical and health personnel in the recognition and management of epilepsy, and to provide information on epilepsy in union publications
11. Urging of national, state, and local voluntary agencies to inform clients of their rights under the Vocational Rehabilitation Act
12. A public health program focusing on employment and epilepsy
13. Development of an employment guide for local communities
14. Making known CETA's "substantial underemployment" areas, in order to encourage more employment opportunities for persons with epilepsy

F. *Job Alternatives:*
1. Adoption of a more effective sheltered workshop compatible for those with epilepsy, for whom conventional employment may not be a realistic solution
2. Pilot projects to investigate the feasibility of employing the severely handicapped within conventional work situations
3. Urging of the National Industries for the Severely Handicapped to provide information to workshops and private groups concerned with epilepsy on services available
4. Permission by the Small Business Administration for nonprofit workshops to bid on contracts in government set-aside programs
5. A general study on the employment of persons with epilepsy in sheltered workshops
6. Identification by voluntary agencies working with the Rehabilitation Service Administration of specific needs for noncompetitive work for persons with epilepsy
7. Congressional enactment of the Wage Supplements for Handicapped Individuals Bill
8. Increasing the work capabilities of persons with epilepsy who are homebound or institutionalized with the help of the Department of Vocational Rehabilitation
9. Legislation by Congress to stipulate that employment, training, and work experience are a part of the "right to treatment" for those who are homebound or institutionalized, making this a priority for Vocational Rehabilitation Innovations and Expansion grants

  10. Identification and promotion of appropriate homebound work areas
G. *Safety:*
  1. Study by the National Institute of Occupational Safety and Health of modifications needed to promote a safe work environment for people subject to seizures
  2. Study of what impact (if any) the employment of persons with epilepsy has on insurance rates
  3. Development and adoption of a model worker's compensation insurance law that includes a uniform second-injury clause to cover employment of persons with epilepsy
  4. Development of guidelines to make schools a safe environment for children with seizures

VI. Independence and Equality
  A. *Minorities:*
    1. Development of public information programs about epilepsy for cultural and minority groups, and inclusion of bilingual personnel and materials in screening and outreach programs
    2. Inclusion by the Developmental Disabilities Office of minority groups in informational and referral programs, minority needs in each state plan, minority representatives on state Developmental Disabilities Councils, and minority access to DD outreach and mobile clinic programs
    3. Assurance of services under Title XX for minorities with epilepsy
    4. Bilingual educational programs on epilepsy in schools in high minority areas
    5. A survey of the presence of persons with developmental disabilities in minority groups
    6. Availability of minority staffing and tax credits for service in minority areas
    7. Production of a glossary of terms used by minorities to describe medical problems
    8. Research on the perception of epilepsy in minority groups
    9. Provision of a list of physicians with cross-cultural experience or a second language
    10. Formation by a nationwide health agency of a committee to focus on minority needs
  B. *Insurance:*
    1. Promotion of group life insurance programs by voluntary groups
    2. Development by the American Bar Association Commission on the Mentally Disabled of model assigned risk

legislation to meet the needs of persons with epilepsy, especially those who are unemployed, and who have been unable to obtain insurance, and enactment of such legislation and initiation of assigned risk programs by the states
3. Preparation of a handbook providing guidance to persons with epilepsy
4. State legislation to make adequate health insurance coverage available to everyone, including those with epilepsy
5. Official studies on the insurability of persons with epilepsy

C. *Financial Assistance:*
1. Congressional reduction of the 24-month waiting period for Medicare benefits to not more than 12 months from the time of original application
2. Making all persons eligible for SSI benefits also eligible for Medicaid in all states
3. Extension of SSI benefits to include Puerto Rico and other U.S. Territories
4. Approved prescription anticonvulsants as a mandated outpatient service under both Medicare and Medicaid
5. Medicare-Medicaid coverage of diagnostic and neurosurgical procedures
6. Maintenance of medical eligibility for assistance under SSI and Social Security Disability Insurance regardless of seizure control until income from other sources offsets program benefits
7. A national study mandated by Congress to determine to what extent persons with epilepsy are a higher health insurance risk than nondisabled persons
8. Examination by Congress of the merits of extending Medicare coverage to persons with epilepsy who do not qualify under the special disability criteria established by Social Security but are unable to obtain private health insurance

D. *Driver's Licensing:*
1. Research into establishing criteria for licensing the driver with epilepsy, with the findings published in the Uniform Motor Vehicle Code and adopted by all the states (at present, licensing conditions for persons with epilepsy vary widely from state to state)
2. Self-reporting of seizure conditions, rather than mandatory reporting by physicians, though the physician should be required to report special patients whom they consider to be a driving hazard
3. Review of license applications by medical advisory boards,

and establishing that licenses *not* be revoked until the individual has had the opportunity to appeal

4. A study of the driving performance of people with epilepsy
5. Permission for high school students with epilepsy who meet state driving requirements to take driver's education, and research on the psychological effect on teenagers who are unable to obtain a driver's license because of epilepsy
6. Adoption of model legislation requiring issuance of an identification card by states for those who cannot be licensed because of epilepsy

E. *Transportation:*

1. Public transportation systems prepared to carry persons with epilepsy, with the necessary built-in safety features for the benefit of those with epilepsy, in accordance with Section 504 of the Vocational Rehabilitation Act
2. Public school transportation for students with epilepsy
3. Increased income tax benefits for volunteer drivers of the handicapped
4. Provision by local volunteers of specific information about the availability of public transportation

F. *Architectural Barriers:*

1. Development of a local complaint procedure by the Architectural Compliance Board, with special attention to the specific needs of people with epilepsy
2. Cooperation between the Occupational Safety and Health Administration and the Architectural Compliance Board to overcome existing gaps
3. A study of the cost and efficacy of removing architectural barriers specific to persons with epilepsy
4. Development of guidance materials for states on how to remove such barriers
5. Monitoring of new and existing public buildings by local epilepsy groups to assure safety of persons subject to seizures

G. *Legal Rights:*

1. Review by state Developmental Disabilities Planning Councils of all relevant federally funded program plans, and congressional expansion of the provisions for the Developmentally Disabled Act to cover all other similar programs, to ensure that the person with epilepsy is not unfairly discriminated against because of the disability
2. Congressional review of Sections 501 through 504 of the Vocational Rehabilitation Act of 1973 and remedial action to ensure their compatibility, and development by other

federal departments of 504 regulations to govern their own programs

3. Congressional amendment of the Civil Rights Act to include the handicapped

4. Amendment of any remaining archaic state laws that permit involuntary sterilization of persons with epilepsy, and mandatory police checks for medical identification before a person with impaired consciousness is taken into custody

5. Efforts by local and national epilepsy groups to inform clients of their rights, to be vigorous advocates on behalf of persons with epilepsy seeking their rights, and to make appropriate statutory changes in states where laws still discriminate against persons with epilepsy

H. *Legal Services:*
 1. The establishment of a clearinghouse with special technical consultation on legal issues affecting those with epilepsy
 2. Development by the American Bar Association Commission on the Mentally Disabled and the National Center for Law and the Handicapped of a program to address specific, unique legal needs of persons with epilepsy
 3. Monitoring of the receipt of services mandated by federal legislation for the handicapped by the Legal Services Corporation
 4. Congressional assurance of the authority of the Department of Justice to protect the constitutional rights of persons in institutions
 5. Publicizing by local epilepsy groups of the availability and means of qualifying for legal services for persons with epilepsy

I. *The Military:*
 1. Examination by the secretaries of the armed forces of existing policies and regulations to permit persons with controlled seizures to serve in the military in selected capacities
 2. Review by the commandants of the Coast Guard and the National Guard of admission and retention policies (including the granting of merchant marine licenses) as they relate to epilepsy, so as to make possible reasonable accommodations in individual situations

VII. Living Arrangements
 A. *Supervised Living Arrangements:*
  1. A census by all the states of people with seizures in all their

residential facilities, with minimum standards of care available in all these facilities

2. A congressionally determined consistency in the standards for institutional care
3. Inclusion by appropriate governmental agencies of regulatory bodies in the medical profession to assure enforcement of the standards of care
4. Adoption of the guidelines by psychiatric facilities serving children

B. *Comprehensive Planning:*
   1. Inclusion in the guidelines for national health planning policy of the philosophy of *one* system of care for all people with epilepsy, wherever they live or whatever services they need
   2. Demonstration by agencies involved in planning as to *how* they will assure a continuum of residential placements, from institutions to foster family or group homes
   3. Testing of community-based model living arrangements
   4. A national demonstration project to collect data and support local planning in this area
   5. Efforts by local epilepsy groups for appropriate zoning ordinances to permit community placement
   6. Publicizing of operating models for smooth de-institutionalization, as examples for others
   7. Respite care provisions in state DD planning

C. *Individual Treatment Plans:*
   1. Development of individual treatment plans (with goals, timetables, and services required) for each institution or residential facility within 10 days of a person's entry, assignment of each plan to a case manager, and inclusion of medical diagnosis and treatment and psychosocial, educational, and vocational needs in these plans

D. *Services:*
   1. Development of collaborative agreements for provision of services between institutions and medical teaching centers and the establishment of ties to the community representative of the Comprehensive Epilepsy Services Network
   2. Provision of adequate medical services for epilepsy to be included in accreditation standards
   3. Assurance that staff of residential facilities serving persons with epilepsy are adequately trained; development of continuing education programs for professional staff
   4. Provision of funds by the Developmental Disabilities Office to allow replication in other parts of the country of a Region

III program that makes university medical services available to institutions with highly favorable results

5. Extension of counseling services for the client and family by state vocational rehabilitation agencies to the institution in order that residents have access to a greater range of vocational opportunities, including noncompetitive employment, and a bill of rights for institutionalized patients with epilepsy

6. An educational plan for each child in an institution to be prepared and followed

E. Community Housing:

1. Amendment of the Social Security Act to avoid the present situation of the institutionalized person's losing much of his SSI benefits, which currently limits the independence of severely handicapped persons with epilepsy, and to permit SSI benefits to be maintained for 90 days if institutionalization is only temporary

2. Publicizing of the opportunities for financing community group living arrangements

3. Efforts by the departments of Housing and Urban Development and Health, Education, and Welfare to provide funding for housing options for persons with epilepsy to avoid unnecessary institutionalization

4. State allocation of funds for needed residential facilities

5. A range of living alternatives to be made available by housing authorities, together with intergovernmental planning committees for the handicapped

6. Maximizing of employment opportunities for the handicapped by local housing authorities

7. Information about rent subsidy eligibility for clients, and advocacy of expanded community housing

F. Correctional Facilities:

1. Making of arrangements with outside providers of medical services to meet the medical needs of prison inmates in accordance with standards of care recommended by the AMA (many prisons, and especially local jails, are not equipped to provide anticonvulsants for inmates with epilepsy)

2. Amendment of the Social Security Act to assure that persons with epilepsy who are arrested and detained do not (as at present) lose the right for reimbursement for medical care

3. When prisoners with epilepsy are discharged, their provi-

sion with a medical plan, medication, and assurance that a
continuing supply of medication will be available

VIII. Education (Patient, Family, Professional, Public)
  A. *Patient and Family:*
      1. Development of specific educational modules about epilep-
         sy, with which the physician could help the person with
         epilepsy and his family realistically to understand his
         potential, seizures, treatment, and possible problem areas
      2. Cooperation between the national voluntary agency con-
         cerned with epilepsy and professional societies to develop
         guidelines and criteria for evaluating the above module
         programs
      3. Compilation by local volunteer groups, working the Com-
         prehensive Epilepsy Programs and the proposed epilepsy
         resource teams, of regional resource directories of available
         services for persons with epilepsy
      4. Development and distribution of a "Guide to Legal Rights
         of Those with Epilepsy"
      5. Testing of family and foster family training programs as to
         value and cost effectiveness
  B. *Physicians:*
      1. As part of their education, providing physicians with a
         basic core of knowledge about epilepsy, with questions on
         epilepsy included in licensing examinations
      2. An increase in the number of clinical fellowships for the
         study of epilepsy
      3. Assignment of medical residents to the proposed Compre-
         hensive Epilepsy Services Network as part of their regular
         medical training
      4. Study by University Affiliated Facilities, which provide
         training to young professionals working in the field of
         developmental disabilities, of their potential role in the
         proposed network; also, development of training programs
         on epilepsy for all levels of medical and allied health
         personnel
      5. Special symposia on the social aspects of epilepsy manage-
         ment
      6. Preparation of materials for use by physicians
      7. Accredited continuing education programs in epilepsy for
         general practitioners, pediatricians, internalists, staffs of
         residential facilities and emergency rooms
      8. Establishment by the proposed National Information Cen-
         ter on Epilepsy of a "consultant hotline" for physicians,

and also production of audiovisual materials on epilepsy for physicians

C. *Obstetricians/Gynecologists:*
1. Symposia to gather material on genetic and obstetrical risks and treatment of epilepsy during pregnancy
2. Preparation of materials focusing on genetic and obstetrical counseling of women with epilepsy for medical schools and similar educational programs

D. *Dentists:*
1. Production of specialized educational materials on the use of anesthetics and on preventative and restorative dental care for persons with epilepsy

E. *Pharmacists:*
1. Educational seminars for pharmacists on the characteristics and use of anticonvulsants
2. A study to involve pharmacists in monitoring the use of anticonvulsants for institutionalized persons with epilepsy
3. A study of the potential role of pharmacists as members of the proposed interdisciplinary epilepsy resource teams
4. Placing materials on anticonvulsants available for publication in pharmaceutical journals

F. *EEG Technologists:*
1. Special training and accreditation standards given to EEG technicians and technologists, according to published guidelines (currently, these professionals are considered by the commission to be receiving inadequate training in epilepsy, in view of the important role the EEG plays in the diagnosis and treatment of epilepsy)

G. *Nurses:*
1. Development of an essential basic curriculum on epilepsy for nurses
2. The addition of nursing programs leading to a clinical specialty in neurological diseases, or a master's degree with expertise in epilepsy
3. Continuing education programs on epilepsy for nurses
4. Questions on epilepsy in certification examinations for RNs and Licensed Practical Nurses
5. The production and dissemination of information on promotion of dental hygiene in patients with epilepsy

H. *Teachers:*
1. A minimum of one course hour in Special Education for the Handicapped, including epilepsy
2. Requirement by certification boards that teaching candidates be able to recognize and assist children who have seizures

      3. Development of training materials on epilepsy for all school and recreational personnel

I. *Social Workers/Counselors:*

      1. Development of programs to train social service personnel in public and private agencies

      2. Regular training sessions on epilepsy for certain vocational rehabilitation counselors

      3. Workshops to develop training materials and addition of this information to the curriculum of graduate and undergraduate schools of rehabilitation studies

      4. Similar training made available to at least one employee in each U.S. Employment Service office

J. *Mental Health Personnel:*

      1. A training program on epilepsy care for community mental health center personnel, developed by the Institute of Mental Health

      2. Development of an information manual on psychological problems of persons with epilepsy, to be distributed throughout the mental health community

K. *Service Personnel:*

      1. Training in recognition and handling of seizures for all public transit (including airline flight) personnel

      2. Materials on seizure recognition and treatment included in police and firefighter training manuals

      3. Special training in epilepsy given to attorneys of local legal service corps, to make them more aware of the needs and legal problems of the handicapped

L. *The Public:*

      1. The development of an active central clearinghouse known as the National Information Center on Epilepsy, initiated by the National Institute of Neurological and Communicative Disorders and Stroke, to collect and store all available public education information materials on epilepsy, develop needed educational materials, and make the information available to the public. The center should work closely with the EFA and other organizations to avoid duplication.

      2. Provision by the American Red Cross of complete and current information on epilepsy in the next revision of its First Aid Manual

IX. Comprehensive Epilepsy Service Network

This network, recommended by the commission, proposes the integration of the network with already existing community resources in an effort to coordinate services at the national level. The system is composed of:

A. *Existing Community Service Providers:*
   private physicians, general practitioners, pediatricians, neurologists, mental health clinics, vocational, recreational, voluntary, and other already existing social service agencies.

B. *Community Resource Person (CRP):*
   a specialist who will work directly with the existing community service providers, providing information and referral, training, and resource development. The CRP is considered the key person "inside" the service system.

C. *Epilepsy Family and Individual Resource Team:*
   a team of persons from several professional disciplines that will provide backup support to the existing community service providers in special problem areas. They will provide training, counseling, and specialized medical and social services, and will conduct clinical research.

D. *Office for Special Neurological Impairments:*
   a federal unit with the responsibility for overseeing and supporting the placement of the Community Resource Persons and the Epilepsy Family and Individual Resource Teams. This office will also guide public and professional education, resource development, quality control, standard setting, and evaluation.

E. *National Information Center on Epilepsy (NICE):*
   a federal office designed to provide current information on epilepsy to those agencies the commission has requested to initiate training on epilepsy for their staffs and other professionals. It will be a central clearinghouse for information on epilepsy and will develop an annual plan for public and professional education, produce audiovisual and printed materials, and support workshops and seminars. The NICE will be administered through the Office for Special Neurological Impairments.

As can readily be seen, these sweeping recommendations by the Commission for the Control of Epilepsy and Its Consequences for the Nationwide Plan should eventually revolutionize the future for all persons with epilepsy, and benefit society in general. If the recommendations are adopted and followed as planned, epilepsy will truly be "out of the closet," and the needless misconceptions and discrimination that have surrounded the disorder for so many centuries will finally be things of the past.

AUTHORS' NOTE

We may not have answered all of your specific questions. Our wish is to help parents and persons with epilepsy to understand and deal with seizure disorders. If you have a question not included in this book, you may send it to us and we will attempt to answer your question or to refer it to someone who can provide either answer or advice. Send questions with a self-addressed stamped envelope to the authors in care of the publisher.

The information regarding federal and state legislation and regulations pertaining to services for epilepsy patients, cited primarily in Chapter 8, is up to date as of June 1981. But government, of course, is never static and changes are inevitable. If you have any questions in regard to public programs your best way to keep abreast of current developments is to contact the specific agency or write your congressman or state representative.

BIBLIOGRAPHY

Aird, R. B., and D. Woodbury. *The Comprehensive Management of Epilepsy.* Springfield, Ill.: Charles C Thomas, Pub., 1974.

Attwell, A. A. *An Outline of Educational Psychology.* Minneapolis: Burgess Publishing Co., 1973.

Bagley, Christopher. *The Social Psychology of the Epileptic Child.* Coral Gables, Fla.: University of Miami Press, 1971.

Baird, H. W. "Convulsive Disorders," in Waldo Nelson, ed., *Textbook of Pediatrics.* Philadelphia: W. B. Saunders Co., 1964.

Basic Statistics on the Epilepsies. Washington, D.C.: Epilepsy Foundation of America, 1975.

Bear, D. M., and P. Fedio. *Quantitative Analysis of Interictal Behavior in Temporal Lobe Epilepsy.* Bethesda, Md.: National Institute of Neurological and Communicative Disorders and Stroke, 1976.

Breger, E., "Attitudinal Survey of Adolescents toward Epileptics of the Same Age Group: Part I, Awareness and Knowledge; Part II, Social Acceptance," *Maryland State Medical Journal* (1976).

Cautela, J., in *B. F. Skinner and Behavior Change.* Film (1975); distributed by Research Press Co., Champaign, Ill.

Chao, D., S. Carter, and A. P. Gold. "Paroxysmal Disorders," in A. Rudolph, ed., *Pediatrics.* New York: Appleton-Century-Crofts, 1977.

Cooper, I. S., M. Riklan, and R. S. Snider. *The Cerebellum, Epilepsy, and Behavior.* New York: Plenum Publishing Corp., 1974.

Gastaut, H. "Clinical Electroencephalographical Classification of Epileptic Seizures," *Epilepsia* 11 (1970).

Gastaut, H., and R. Broughton. *Epileptic Seizures: Clinical and Electrographic Features, Diagnosis and Treatment.* Springfield, Ill.: Charles C Thomas, Pub., 1972.

Gunn, J. "The Prevalence of Epilepsy in Prisoners," *Journal of the Royal Society of Medicine* 62 (1969): 60–63.

Hauser, W. A., and L. T. Kurland. "The Epidemiology of Epilepsy in Rochester, Minnesota, 1935 through 1967," *Epilepsia* 16 (1975).

Henriksen, B., P. Juul-Jensen, and M. Lund. "The Mortality of Epileptics," in *Proceedings*, Tenth International Congress on Life Assurance Medicine. London: Pilsmen Co. Ltd., 1970.

Holowach, J., D. Thurston, and J. O'Leary. "Prognosis in Childhood Epilepsy: Follow-up Study," *New England Journal of Medicine* 286 (1972).

King, L., and Q. Young. "Increased Prevalence of Seizure Disorders among Prisoners," *Journal of the American Medical Association* 239 (June 23, 1978).

Laidlaw, J., and A. Richens. *A Textbook of Epilepsy.* New York: Churchill Livingstone, 1976.

Lennox, W. G., and M. A. Lennox. *Epilepsy and Related Disorders.* Boston: Little, Brown & Co., 1960.

Livingston, S. *Comprehensive Management of Epilepsy in Infancy, Childhood and Adolescence.* Springfield, Ill.: Charles C Thomas, Pub., 1971.

———. "Psychosocial Aspects of Epilepsy," *Journal of Clinical Child Psychology* 6 (1977).

Lombroso, C. T. "The Treatment of Status Epilepticus," *Pediatrics* 53 (1974).

Lubar, J., and W. Bahler. "Behavioral Management of Epileptic Seizures Following EEG Biofeedback Training of Sensorimotor Rhythm," *Biofeedback and Self-Regulation* 1 (1976): 77–104.

Masland, R., et al. *Plan for Nationwide Action on Epilepsy.* Washington, D.C.: U.S. Department of Health, Education, and Welfare, 1977.

Meighan, S., L. Queener, and M. Weitman. "Prevalence of Epilepsy in Children of Multnomah County, Oregon," *Epilepsia* 17 (1976): 245–256.

Metrakos, J. D., and K. Metrakos. "Genetic Studies in Clinical Epilepsy," in H. Jasper et al., *Basic Mechanics of the Epilepsies.* Boston: Little, Brown & Co., 1969.

Millichap, J. G. *Febrile Convulsions.* New York: Macmillan Publishing Co., 1968.

Niedermeyer, E. *Compendium on the Epilepsies.* Springfield, Ill.: Charles C Thomas, Pub., 1974.

Ornstein, Robert. *The Psychology of Consciousness.* New York: Penguin Books, 1975.

Ovellette, E. M. "The Child who Convulses with Fever," *Pediatric Clinics of North America* 21 (1974).

Penfield, W., and H. Jasper. *Epilepsy and the Functional Anatomy of the Human Brain.* Boston: Little, Brown & Co., 1954.

Perlman, L., and L. Strudler. "Unfair Insurance Practices Concerning Epilepsy." Testimony before the Unfair Discrimination Hearings on Insurance. Philadelphia, February 19, 1975.

Rose, S. W., et al. "Prevalence of Epilepsy in Children," *Epilepsia* 14 (1973).

Schmidt, R. P., and B. J. Wilder. *Epilepsy.* Philadelphia: F. A. Davis Co., 1968.

Wilder, J. *The Clinical Neurophysiology of Epilepsy: A Survey of Current Research.* Washington, D.C.: U.S. Department of Health, Education, and Welfare, 1968.

A

DIRECTORIES, GOVERNMENT ORGANIZATIONS, COMPREHENSIVE EPILEPSY PROGRAMS, NATIONAL ORGANIZATIONS

DIRECTORIES

Directory of Association of Rehabilitation Facilities (1978)
Publications Department, Association of Rehabilitation Services
5530 Wisconsin Avenue, Suite 955
Washington, DC 20201
Free

Directory of Educational Facilities for the Learning Disabled (1979–1980)
Association for Children with Learning Disabilities
4156 Library Road
Pittsburgh, PA 15234
$1.50

Directory for Exceptional Children (1978)
Porter Sargent Publishers, Inc.
11 Beacon Street
Boston, MA 02108
$25

Directory of Homemaker–Home Health Aid Services (1980)

National Council for Homemaker Services, Inc.
67 Irving Place
New York, NY 10003
$10

Directory of Inpatient Facilities for the Mentally Retarded (1975)
U.S. Government Printing Office
Washington, DC 20402
$2.85

Directory of Organizations Interested in the Handicapped (1980)
People to People Committee for the Handicapped
1522 K Street NW
Washington, DC 20005
$2 to handicapped individuals or their families

Directory of Private Schools for Exceptional Children (1977)
National Association of Private Schools for Exceptional Children
P.O. Box 928
Lake Wales, FL 33853
Single copy free

Directory for Special Children (1975)
American Association of Special
  Educators
P.O. Box 168
Fryeburg, ME 04037
$5

*Directory of State Divisions of
  Vocational Rehabilitation* (1978)
U.S. Rehabilitation Services
  Administration, Social and
  Rehabilitation Service
330 C Street SW
Washington, DC 20201
Free

*Directory of Summer Camps for
  Children with Learning Disabilities*
  (1974)
Association for Children with
  Learning Disabilities
5225 Grace Street
Pittsburgh, PA 15236
$1.25

*Easter Seal Directory of Resident
  Camps for Persons with Special
  Health Needs* (1977)
National Easter Seal Society for
  Crippled Children and Adults
2023 West Ogden Avenue
Chicago, IL 60612
$2

*Guide for Clinical Services in Speech
  Pathology and Audiology* (1977)
American Speech and Hearing
  Association
9030 Old Georgetown Road
Washington, DC 20014
$10

Guide to Epilepsy Services (1978)
Epilepsy Foundation of America
4351 Garden City Drive
Landover, MD 20785
Single copy and individual state
  pages free

Mental Health Directory (1976)
National Institutes of Mental
  Health
SN 017–024–00489–8
U.S. Government Printing Office
Washington, DC 20402
$6.50

*Residential Facilities for the
  Handicapped*
Closer Look: National Information
  Center for the Handicapped
Box 1492
Washington, DC 20013

GOVERNMENT ORGANIZATIONS

National Institute of Neurological
  and Communicative Disorders
  and Stroke

Office of Public Affairs, Building
  31
9000 Rockville Pike
Bethesda, MD 20205

To locate the agency that serves the *developmentally disabled* in your
area, contact the office of developmental disabilities in your state:

ALABAMA
Dept. of Mental Health
Developmental Disabilities
  Program
502 Washington Street
Montgomery, AL 36130
(205) 265-2301

ALASKA
Dept. of Health and Social
  Services
Developmental Disabilities
  Program
Division of Mental Health
Pouch H-04B

Juneau, AK 99801
(907) 465-3372

ARIZONA
State Dept. of Economic Security
Developmental Disabilities
  Program
P.O. Box 6123
Phoenix, AZ 85005
(602) 271-5678

ARKANSAS
Dept. of Social and Rehabilitative
  Services
Developmental Disabilities
  Program
Waldon Avenue Bldg., Suite 400
7th and Main Streets
Little Rock, AR 72201
(501) 371-3482

CALIFORNIA
Dept. of Developmental Services
Program Development Section
Developmental Disabilities
  Program
744 P Street
Sacramento, CA 95814
(916) 920-6795

COLORADO
Dept. of Institutions
Division of Developmental
  Disabilities
4150 South Lowell Boulevard
Denver, CO 80236
(303) 761-0220

CONNECTICUT
Dept. of Mental Retardation
Developmental Disabilities
  Program
79 Elm Street
Hartford, CT 06115
(203) 566-2034

DELAWARE
Dept. of Health and Social
  Services

Developmental Disabilities
  Program
3000 Newport Gap Pike
Wilmington, DE 19808
(302) 421-6705

DISTRICT OF COLUMBIA
Dept. of Human Resources
Developmental Disabilities
  Program
1329 E Street NW, Room 1023
Washington, DC 20004
(202) 724-4696

FLORIDA
Dept. of Health and Rehabilitative
  Services
Division of Retardation
Developmental Disabilities
  Program
1311 Winewood Boulevard
Tallahassee, FL 32301
(904) 488-4257

GEORGIA
Dept. of Human Resources
Division of Mental Health and
  Mental Retardation
Developmental Disabilities
  Program
47 Trinity Avenue, SW, Room
  542-H
Atlanta, GA 30334
(404) 656-6370

HAWAII
State Dept. of Health
Developmental Disabilities
  Program
P.O. Box 3378
Honolulu, HI 96801
(808) 548-6506, 6-0220

IDAHO
Dept. of Health and Welfare

Division of Community
  Rehabilitation
Developmental Disabilities
  Program
State House
Boise, ID 83720
(208) 384-3920

ILLINOIS
Dept. of Mental Health
Developmental Disabilities
  Program
401 South Spring Street
Springfield, IL 62706
(217) 782-2243

INDIANA
Dept. of Mental Health
5 Indiana Square
Indianapolis, IN 46204
(317) 633-7562

IOWA
Office for Planning and Programs
Developmental Disabilities
  Program
523 East 12th Street
Des Moines, IA 50319
(515) 281-5880

KANSAS
Dept. of Social and Rehabilitation
  Services
Developmental Disabilities
  Program
State Office Building — Sixth Floor
Topeka, KS 66612
(913) 296-3471

KENTUCKY
Bureau for Health Services
Developmental Disabilities
  Program
275 East Main Street
Frankfort, KY 40601
(502) 564-7190

LOUISIANA
Health and Human Resources
  Administration
Division of Mental Retardation
Developmental Disabilities
  Program
P.O. Box 44215
Baton Rouge, LA 70802
(504) 389-2360

MAINE
Dept. of Mental Health and
  Correction
Bureau of Mental Retardation
Developmental Disabilities
  Program
State Office Building Room 411
Augusta, ME 04330
(207) 289-3167

MARYLAND
Dept. of Health and Mental
  Hygiene
301 West Preston Street
Baltimore, MD 21201
(301) 383-3358

MASSACHUSETTS
Administrative Agency for
  Developmental Disabilities
1 Ashburton Place
Boston, MA 02113
(617) 727-4178

MICHIGAN
Dept. of Mental Health
Developmental Disabilities
  Program
Lewis-Cass Building
Lansing, MI 48926
(517) 373-3500

MINNESOTA
State Planning Agency
Developmental Disabilities
  Program
200 Capitol Square Building

550 Cedar Street
St. Paul, MN 55101
(612) 296–4018

MISSISSIPPI
Dept. of Mental Health
Division of Mental Retardation
Developmental Disabilities
    Program
1404 Woolfolk Building
Jackson, MS 39201
(601) 354–6692

MISSOURI
Dept. of Mental Health
Developmental Disabilities
    Program
2002 Missouri Boulevard, P.O.
    Box 687
Jefferson City, MO 65101
(314) 751–4054

MONTANA
Dept. of Social and Rehabilitation
    Services
Developmental Disabilities
    Program
507 Power Block
Helena, MT 59601
(406) 449–2995

NEBRASKA
Dept. of Health
Developmental Disabilities
    Program
P.O. Box 95007
Lincoln, NB 68509
(402) 471–2981

NEVADA
Dept. of Human Resources
Developmental Disabilities
    Program
600 Kinkead Building, Capitol
    Complex
Carson City, NV 89710
(702) 885–4730

NEW HAMPSHIRE
Dept. of Health and Welfare
Division of Mental Health
Office of Mental Retardation
Developmental Disabilities
    Program
105 Pleasant Street
Concord, NH 03301
(603) 842–2671

NEW JERSEY
Office of Human Services
Division of Mental Retardation
Developmental Disabilities
    Program
169 West Hanover Street
Trenton, NJ 08625
(609) 292–3742

NEW MEXICO
Dept. of Education
Division of Vocational
    Rehabilitation
Developmental Disabilities
    Program
P.O. Box 1830
Santa Fe, NM 87503
(505) 476–2266

NEW YORK
Office of Mental Retardation and
    Developmental Disabilities
Developmental Disabilities
    Program
44 Holland Avenue
Albany, NY 12203
(518) 474–6566

NORTH CAROLINA
Developmental Disabilities Council
    Staff
3225 North Salisbury Street, Room
    612
Raleigh, NC 27611
(919) 733–7787

NORTH DAKOTA
Dept. of Health

Division of Mental Health and
 Mental Retardation
Developmental Disabilities
 Program
909 Basin Avenue
Bismarck, ND 58505
(701) 224-2769

OHIO
Dept. of Mental Health and
 Mental Retardation
Developmental Disabilities
 Program
30 East Broad Street, Room 1182
Columbus, OH 43215
(614) 466-5205

OKLAHOMA
Dept. of Institutions, Social and
 Rehabilitation Services
Developmental Disabilities
 Program
P.O. Box 25352
Oklahoma City, OK 73125
(405) 521-3617

OREGON
Dept. of Mental Retardation and
 Developmental Disabilities
Mental Health Division
Developmental Disabilities
 Program
2575 Bittern Street, NE
Salem, OR 97310
(503) 378-2429

PENNSYLVANIA
Office of Human Resources
Developmental Disabilities
 Program
900 Market Street
Harrisburg, PA 17105
(717) 787-3409

RHODE ISLAND
Dept. of Mental Health,
 Retardation and Hospitals

Developmental Disabilities
 Program
Aime J. Forand Building
600 New London Avenue
Cranston, RI 02920
(401) 464-3231

SOUTH CAROLINA
Office of the Governor
Division of Administration
Developmental Disabilities
 Program
Edgar Brown Building, Room 408
1205 Pendleton Street
Columbia, SC 29240
(803) 758-7886

SOUTH DAKOTA
Division of Mental Health and
 Mental Retardation
Dept. of Social Services
Developmental Disabilities
 Program
State Office Building, Third Floor
Pierre, SD 57501
(605) 224-3438

TENNESSEE
Dept. of Mental Health and
 Mental Retardation
Developmental Disabilities
 Program
501 Union Building, Fourth Floor
Nashville, TN 37219
(615) 741-3803

TEXAS
Dept. of Mental Health and
 Mental Retardation
Developmental Disabilities
 Program
Box 12668, Capitol Station
Austin, TX 78711
(512) 454-3761

UTAH
Division of Family Services

Developmental Disabilities
Program
150 West North Temple, Suite 370
Salt Lake City, UT 84103
(801) 533–7127

VERMONT
Agency of Human Services
Developmental Disabilities
Program
79 River Street
Montpelier, VT 05602
(802) 828–2471

VIRGINIA
Dept. of Mental Health and
Mental Retardation
Developmental Disabilities
Program
109 Governor Street, P.O. Box
1797
Richmond, VA 23214
(840) 770–4982

WASHINGTON
Dept. of Social and Health
Services
Developmental Disabilities
Program
P.O. Box 1162

Olympia, WA 98501
(206) 434–3900

WEST VIRGINIA
Dept. of Mental Health and
Mental Retardation
Developmental Disabilities
Program
State Capitol
Charleston, WV 25305
(304) 348–2971

WISCONSIN
Dept. of Health and Social
Services
Developmental Disabilities
Program
1 West Wilson Street
Madison, WI 53702
(608) 266–3304

WYOMING
Dept. of Health and Social
Services
Division of Mental Health/Mental
Retardation
Developmental Disabilities
Program
State Office Building West
Cheyenne, WY 82001
(307) 777–7115

To locate the nearest program for *crippled or handicapped children* in your area, contact your local board of health, or the office for crippled or handicapped children in your state:

ALABAMA
Crippled Children's Services
2129 East South Blvd.
Montgomery, AL 36111
(205) 281–8780

ALASKA
State Dept. of Health and Social
Services
Family Health Section

Pouch H, Health and Welfare
Building
Juneau, AK 99801
(907) 465–3100

ARIZONA
State Crippled Children's Hospital
200 North Curry Road
Tempe, AZ 85281
(602) 244–9471

ARKANSAS
Dept. of Social and Rehabilitative
  Services
Arkansas Social Services
Crippled Children's Section
P.O. Box 1437
Little Rock, AR 72203
(501) 371-2277

CALIFORNIA
State Dept. of Health
Crippled Children's Services
  Section
741-744 P Street
Sacramento, CA 95814
(916) 322-2090

COLORADO
Dept. of Health
Handicapped Children's Program
4210 East Eleventh Avenue
Denver, CO 80220
(303) 388-6111

CONNECTICUT
State Dept. of Health
Crippled Children's Section
79 Elm Street
Hartford, CT 06115
(203) 566-5425

DELAWARE
Bureau of Personal Health Services
Division of Public Health
Jesse Cooper Memorial Building
Capital Square
Dover, DE 19901
(302) 678-4768

DISTRICT OF COLUMBIA
Dept. of Human Resources
Maternal and Child Health and
  Crippled Children's Services
1875 Connecticut Ave. NW
Washington, DC 20001
(202) 673-6670

FLORIDA
Dept. of Health and Rehabilitative
  Services
Children's Medical Services
  Program
Building 5, 1323 Winewood Blvd.
Tallahassee, FL 32301
(904) 487-2690

GEORGIA
Dept. of Human Resources
Division of Physical Health
Crippled Children's Unit
618 Ponce de Leon Ave. NE
Atlanta, GA 30308
(404) 894-4081

HAWAII
State Dept. of Health
Crippled Children's Services
P.O. Box 3378
Honolulu, HI 96801
(808) 548-5830

IDAHO
State Dept. of Health and Welfare
Bureau of Child Health
Crippled Children's Services
State House
700 West State Street
Boise, ID 83720
(208) 384-2136

ILLINOIS
Division of Services for Crippled
  Children
540 Iles Park Place
Springfield, IL 62718
(217) 782-7001

INDIANA
State Dept. of Public Welfare
Division of Services for Crippled
  Children, Room 702
100 North Senate Avenue
Indianapolis, IN 46204
(317) 232-4280

IOWA
State Services for Crippled
  Children
University of Iowa
Iowa City, IA 52242
(319) 353–4431

KANSAS
State Dept. of Health and
  Environment
Bureau of Maternal and Child
  Health
Topeka, KS 66620
(913) 862–9360 ext. 437

KENTUCKY
State Dept. of Human Resources
Bureau for Health Services
275 East Main Street
Frankfort, KY 40601
(502) 564–4830

LOUISIANA
Dept. of Health and Human
  Resources
Handicapped Children's Program
P.O. Box 60630
New Orleans, LA 70160
(504) 568–5048

MAINE
Division of Child Health
Dept. of Human Resources
State House
Augusta, ME 04330
(207) 289–3311

MARYLAND
Dept. of Health and Mental
  Hygiene
Preventative Medicine
  Administration
Division of Crippled Children
201 West Preston Street
Baltimore, MD 21201
(301) 383–2821

MASSACHUSETTS
State Dept. of Public Health
Division of Family Health
39 Boylston Street
Boston, MA 02116
(617) 737–3372

MICHIGAN
Dept. of Public Health
Bureau of Personal Health
  Services
3500 North Logan Street
Lansing, MI 48914
(517) 373–3650

MINNESOTA
Dept. of Health
Crippled Children's Services
717 Delaware Street SE
Minneapolis, MN 55440
(612) 296–5372

MISSISSIPPI
State Board of Health
Bureau of Family Health Services
Crippled Children's Services
P.O. Box 1700
Jackson, MS 39205
(601) 354–6680

MISSOURI
Dept. of Social Services
Division of Health
Crippled Children's Services
P.O. Box 570, Third Floor
Broadway State Office Building
Jefferson City, MO 65101
(314) 751–4667

MONTANA
Dept. of Health and Environment
  Sciences
Health Services Division
Maternal and Child Health
Cogswell Building
Helena, MT 59601
(405) 449–2554

NEBRASKA
Dept. of Public Welfare
Services for Crippled Children
301 Centennial Mall, Fifth Floor
Lincoln, NB 68509
(402) 471–3121 ext. 186

NEVADA
State Dept. of Human Resources
Division of Public Health
505 East King Street
Room 205, Capital Complex
Carson City, NV 89701
(702) 885–4885

NEW HAMPSHIRE
State Dept. of Health and Welfare
Division of Public Health
61 South Spring Street
Concord, NH 03301
(603) 842–2681

NEW JERSEY
State Dept. of Health
Crippled Children's Program
Health and Agricultural Building
Trenton, NJ 08625
(609) 292–5676

NEW MEXICO
Health and Social Services Dept.
Office of Family Services
P.O. Box 2348
Santa Fe, NM 87501
(505) 827–3201

NEW YORK
State Dept. of Health
Bureau of Medical Rehabilitation
Empire State Plaza
Tower Building
Albany, NY 12237
(518) 474–1911

NORTH CAROLINA
Dept. of Human Resources
Crippled Children's Section
Division of Health Services

P.O. Box 2091
Raleigh, NC 27602
(919) 733–7437

NORTH DAKOTA
Social Service Board
State Capitol Building
Bismarck, ND 58501
(701) 224–2436

OHIO
State Dept. of Health
Division of Maternal and Child
  Health
P.O. Box 118
450 East Town Street
Columbus, OH 43215
(614) 466–3263

OKLAHOMA
Dept. of Institutions, Social and
  Rehabilitative Services
Crippled Children's Unit
P.O. Box 25352
Oklahoma City, OK 73125
(405) 271–3902

OREGON
Crippled Children's Division
University of Oregon Medical
  School
3181 Southwest Sam Jackson Park
  Road
Portland, OR 97201
(503) 225–8362

PENNSYLVANIA
State Dept. of Health
Bureau of Children's Services
Children's Rehabilitation Services
407 South Cameron Street
Harrisburg, PA 17120
(717) 783–5436

RHODE ISLAND
Dept. of Health
Division of Child Health
75 Davis Street, Room 302

Providence, RI 02908
(401) 277–2312

SOUTH CAROLINA
Dept. of Health and
  Environmental Control
Children's Services
J. Marion Sims Building
Columbia, SC 29201
(803) 758–5594

SOUTH DAKOTA
State Dept. of Health
Division of Health Services
Foss Building
Pierre, SD 57501
(605) 224–3141

TENNESSEE
State Dept. of Public Health
Crippled Children's Services
347 Cordell Hull Building
Nashville, TN 37219
(615) 741–7335

TEXAS
Dept. of Health
Crippled Children's Program
1100 West 49th Street
Austin, TX 78576
(512) 458–7700

UTAH
State Division of Health
Crippled Children's Services
44 Medical Drive
Salt Lake City, UT 84113
(801) 533–4390

VERMONT
Dept. of Health
Child Health Services
115 Colchester Avenue
Burlington, VT 05402
(802) 862–5701 ext. 311

VIRGINIA
State Dept. of Health
Division of Hospital Medical
  Services
Bureau of Crippled Children's
  Services
109 Governor Street
Richmond, VA 23219
(804) 770–3691

WASHINGTON
Dept. of Social and Health
  Services
Division of Health Services
Child Health Section MS:
  LC-12-A
Olympia, WA 98504
(206) 753–2571

WEST VIRGINIA
State Dept. of Welfare
Division of Crippled Children's
  Services
1212 Lewis Street, Morris Square
Charleston, WV 25301
(304) 348–3071

WISCONSIN
State Dept. of Public Instruction
Bureau for Crippled Children
126 Langdon Street
Madison, WI 53702
(608) 266–3886

WYOMING
State Dept. of Health and Social
  Services
Division of Health and Medical
  Services
Hathaway Office Building
Cheyenne, WY 82002
(307) 777–7121

For information and assistance in obtaining *special education services*, contact your local school district, or the office of special education in your state:

ALABAMA
State Dept. of Education
Exceptional Children and Youth
868 State Office Building
Montgomery, AL 36104
(205) 832-3230

ALASKA
State Dept. of Education
Exceptional Children and Youth
  Section
Division of Instructional Services
Pouch F
Juneau, AK 99801
(907) 465-2970

ARIZONA
State Dept. of Education
Special Education Division
1535 West Jefferson
Phoenix, AZ 85007
(602) 255-5198

ARKANSAS
State Dept. of Education
Division of Instructional Services
Arch Ford Education Building
Little Rock, AR 72201
(501) 371-2161

CALIFORNIA
Dept. of Special Education
Public Instruction
721 Capitol Mall, Room 614
Sacramento, CA 95814
(916) 445-4036

COLORADO
State Dept. of Education
Pupil Services Unit
State Office Building
201 East Colfax Avenue
Denver, CO 80203
(303) 839-2727

CONNECTICUT
State Dept. of Education
Division of Student Services
Box 2219

Hartford, CT 06115
(203) 566-4383

DELAWARE
State Dept. of Public Instruction
Townsend Building
Dover, DE 19901
(302) 678-5471

DISTRICT OF COLUMBIA
Board of Education
Division of Special Educational
  Programs
415 Twelfth Street NW
Washington, DC 20004
(202) 724-4018

FLORIDA
State Dept. of Education
Bureau of Education for
  Exceptional Students
Tallahassee, FL 32304
(904) 488-1570 or 488-3205

GEORGIA
Dept. of Education
Program for Exceptional Children
State Office Building
Atlanta, GA 30334
(404) 656-2678

HAWAII
Dept. of Education
Special Needs Branch
Box 2360
Honolulu, HI 96804
(808) 548-6923

IDAHO
State Dept. of Education
Special Education Division
Len Jordan Building
Boise, ID 83720
(208) 384-2203

ILLINOIS
Dept. of Education
Dept. of Special Educational
  Services

100 North First Street
Springfield, IL 62777
(217) 782–6601

INDIANA
State Dept. of Public Instruction
Division of Special Education
229 State House
Indianapolis, IN 46204
(317) 927–0216

IOWA
State Dept. of Public Instruction
Division of Special Education
Grimes State Office Building
Des Moines, IA 50319
(515) 281–3176

KANSAS
State Dept. of Education
Division of Special Education
120 East Tenth Street
Topeka, KS 66612
(913) 296–3866

KENTUCKY
Bureau of Education for
  Exceptional Children
Capitol Plaza Tower - Eighth Floor
Frankfort, KY 40601
(502) 564–4970

LOUISIANA
State Dept. of Education
Special Education Services
P.O. Box 44064 Capitol Station
Baton Rouge, LA 70804
(504) 342–3641

MAINE
State Dept. of Education and
  Cultural Services
Division of Special Education
Augusta, ME 04330
(207) 289–3451

MARYLAND
State Dept. of Education
Division of Special Education

P.O. Box 8717, BWI Airport
Baltimore, MD 21240
(301) 796–8300 ext. 256

MASSACHUSETTS
State Dept. of Education
Division of Special Education
31 St. James Avenue
Boston, MA 02116
(617) 727–6217

MICHIGAN
State Dept. of Education
Special Education Services
P.O. Box 420
Lansing, MI 48902
(517) 373–1695

MINNESOTA
State Dept. of Education
Special Education Section
Capitol Square, 550 Cedar Street
St. Paul, MN 55101
(612) 296–4163

MISSISSIPPI
State Dept. of Education
Division of Special Education
P.O. Box 771
Jackson, MS 39205
(601) 354–6950

MISSOURI
Dept. of Elementary and
  Secondary Education
Division of Special Education
P.O. Box 480
Jefferson City, MO 65101
(314) 751–2965

MONTANA
Office for the Superintendent of
  Public Instruction
Division of Special Education
State Capitol
Helena, MT 59601
(406) 449–5660

NEBRASKA
State Dept. of Education
Special Education Section
223 South Tenth Street
Lincoln, NB 68508
(402) 471–2471

NEVADA
State Dept. of Education
Division of Special Education
400 W. King Street - Capitol
 Complex
Carson City, NV 89701
(702) 885–5700 ext. 214

NEW HAMPSHIRE
State Dept. of Education
Special Education
105 Loudon Road, Building 3
Concord, NH 03301
(603) 271–3741

NEW JERSEY
State Dept. of Education
225 West State Street
Trenton, NJ 08625
(609) 292–7602

NEW MEXICO
State Dept. of Education
Division of Special Education
State Education Building
300 Don Gaspar Avenue
Santa Fe, NM 87503
(505) 872–2793

NEW YORK
State Dept. of Education
Office for Education of Children
 with Handicapping Conditions
55 Elk Street
Albany, NY 12234
(518) 474–5548

NORTH CAROLINA
State Dept. of Public Instruction
Division for Exceptional Children
Raleigh, NC 27611
(919) 733–3921

NORTH DAKOTA
State Dept. of Public Instruction
Special Education
Bismarck, ND 58501
(701) 224–2277

OHIO
State Dept. of Education
Division of Special Education
933 High Street
Worthington, OH 43085
(614) 466–2650

OKLAHOMA
State Dept. of Education
Division of Special Education
2500 N. Lincoln, Suite 263
Oklahoma City, OK 73105
(405) 521–3351

OREGON
State Dept. of Education
Division of Special Education
942 Lancaster Drive, NE
Salem, OR 97310
(503) 378–3598

PENNSYLVANIA
State Dept. of Education
Bureau of Special and
 Compensatory Education
P.O. Box 911
Harrisburg, PA 17126
(717) 783–1264

RHODE ISLAND
State Dept. of Education
Division of Special Education
235 Promenade Street
Providence, RI 02908
(401) 277–3505

SOUTH CAROLINA
State Dept. of Education
Office of Programs for the
 Handicapped
Room 309, Rutledge Building
Columbia, SC 29201
(803) 758–7432

SOUTH DAKOTA
Division of Elementary and
Secondary Education
Section for Special Education
New State Office Building
Pierre, SD 57501
(606) 773-3678

TENNESSEE
State Dept. of Education
Education of the Handicapped
103 Cordell Hull Building
Nashville, TN 37219
(615) 741-2851

TEXAS
Education Agency
Division of Special Education
201 East Eleventh Street
Austin, TX 78701
(512) 475-3501 or 475-3507

UTAH
State Board of Education
Pupil Services Coordinator
250 East 5th Street
Salt Lake City, UT 84111
(801) 533-5982

VERMONT
State Dept. of Education
Special Education and Pupil
Personnel Services
Montpelier, VT 05602
(802) 828-3141

VIRGINIA
State Dept. of Education
Division of Special Education
322 E. Grace
Richmond, VA 23216
(804) 786-2673

WASHINGTON
Dept. of Pupil Instruction
Special and Institutional
Education
Old Capitol Building
Olympia, WA 98504
(206) 753-2563

WEST VIRGINIA
State Dept. of Education
Division of Special Education
Student Support System
Capitol Complex — B-057
Charleston, WV 25305
(304) 348-2034

WISCONSIN
State Dept. of Public Instruction
Division for Handicapped Children
126 Langdon Street
Madison, WI 53702
(608) 266-1649

WYOMING
State Dept. of Education
Office of Exceptional Children
Cheyenne, WY 82002
(307) 777-7416

COMPREHENSIVE EPILEPSY PROGRAMS

CALIFORNIA
Department of Neurology
UCLA Center for Health Control
Los Angeles, CA 90024
(213) 824-4303

GEORGIA
Department of Neurology

Medical College of Georgia
Augusta, GA 30901
(404) 828-4533

MINNESOTA
University of Minnesota
2829 University Avenue S.E., Suite
608

Minneapolis, MN 55414
(612) 376–5031
OREGON
Good Samaritan Hospital and
 Medical Center
2222 N.W. Lovejoy, Suite 361
Portland, OR 97210
(503) 229–7220
VIRGINIA
University of Virginia Medical

Center, Box 403
Charlottesville, VA 22901
(804) 924–5401

WASHINGTON
Epilepsy Center at Harborview
325 Ninth Avenue
Seattle, WA 98104
(206) 233–3573

ORGANIZATIONS

Association for Children with
 Learning Disabilities
4156 Library Road
Pittsburgh, PA 15234

Association for Retarded Citizens
National Headquarters
2501 Avenue J
Arlington, TX 76011

Closer Look
National Information Center

Box 1492
Washington, DC 20013

National Easter Seal Society for
 Crippled Children and Adults
2023 West Ogden Avenue
Chicago, IL 60612

Epilepsy Foundation of America
4351 Garden City Drive
Landover, MD 20785
(301) 459–3700

There are usually several affiliates of the EFA in each state; the following list
gives the major one. Addresses and telephone numbers may change, so we
recommend that you call or write the EFA at the Maryland number and
address above if you have any problem obtaining information in your state.

ALABAMA
Epilepsy Chapter of Mobile and
 Gulf Coast
951 Government Street, Suite 116
Mobile, AL 36604
(205) 432–0970

ALASKA
Anchorage Area Epilepsy Society
P.O. Box 24933
Anchorage, AK 99509
(907) 274–3862

ARIZONA
Central Arizona Regional Epilepsy
 Society
1802 East Thomas Road No. 13
Phoenix, AZ 85016
(602) 279–5721

ARKANSAS
Arkansas Epilepsy Society, Inc.
4120 West Markham Street, Suite
 101
Little Rock, AR 72201
(501) 666–1355

CALIFORNIA
California Epilepsy Society
6117 Reseda Boulevard, Suite G
Reseda, CA 91335
(213) 342–1709

COLORADO
Colorado Epilepsy Association
1835 Gaylord Street
Denver, CO 80206
(303) 321–3266

CONNECTICUT
Southern Connecticut Epilepsy
  Foundation
165 Ocean Terrace
Bridgeport, CT 06605
(203) 334–0854

DELAWARE
Delaware Epilepsy Association
2705 Baynard Boulevard
Wilmington, DE 19802
(302) 658–9847

DISTRICT OF COLUMBIA
Washington DC Area Chapter
815 Fifteenth Street NW, Suite 706
Washington, DC 20005
(202) 638–5229

FLORIDA
The Council on Epilepsy
230 Rawls Avenue
Sarasota, FL 33577
(813) 953–5988

GEORGIA
Georgia Chapter, EFA
57 Forsyth Street NW
Atlanta, GA 30303
(404) 523–4197

HAWAII
Hawaii Epilepsy Society
200 North Vineyard Boulevard

Honolulu, HI 96817
(808) 523–7705

IDAHO
Idaho Epilepsy League
750 Warm Springs Avenue, Suite
  B
Boise, ID 93702
(208) 344–4340

ILLINOIS
Midwest Epilepsy Center
929 South Main Street
Lombard, IL 60148
(312) 627–6445

INDIANA
Tri-State Epilepsy Association
421 North Main Street
Evansville, IN 47711
(812) 426–1451

IOWA
Iowa Chapter, EFA
c/o Rob Riley
621 Ovid Avenue
Des Moines, IA 50313
(515) 281–1548 or 347–8421

KANSAS
Kansas Chapter, EFA
2721 Boulevard Plaza
Wichita, KS 67211
(316) 684–0591

KENTUCKY
Epilepsy Association of Kentucky,
  Inc.
845 Lane Allen Road, Suite 14
Lexington, KY 40504
(606) 278–5472

LOUISIANA
Louisiana Epilepsy Association
200 Medical Center
4550 North Boulevard
Baton Rouge, LA 70806
(504) 928–4482

MAINE
Pinetree Epilepsy Association
622 Congress Street
Portland, ME 04101
(207) 772-7847

MARYLAND
Epilepsy Association of Maryland
3121 St. Paul Street, Suite 20
Baltimore, MD 21218
(301) 243-4811

MASSACHUSETTS
Epilepsy Support Program
c/o Emerson Hospital
Concord, MA 01742
(617) 369-1460

MICHIGAN
Epilepsy Center of Michigan
3800 Woodward, Seventh Floor
Professional Plaza
Detroit, MI 48201
(313) 832-0500

MINNESOTA
Minnesota Epilepsy League
Citizens Aid Building Room 242
404 South Eighth Street
Minneapolis, MN 55404
(612) 340-7630

MISSISSIPPI
Mississippi Council on Epilepsy
3000 Old Canton Road, Suite 470
Jackson, MS 39216
(601) 362-2761

MISSOURI
Greater Kansas City Epilepsy
  League
4049 Pennsylvania, Room 208
Kansas City, MO 64111
(816) 531-1247

MONTANA
Butte Epilepsy Association
P.O. Box 4012
Butte, MT 59701
(406) 723-4243

NEBRASKA
Nebraska Epilepsy League, Inc.
3610 Dodge Street, No. 201
Omaha, NB 68131
(402) 342-0290

NEVADA
Southern Nevada Epilepsy Society
1000 South Third, Suite C
Las Vegas, NV 89101
(702) 384-2393 (C. Brown)

NEW JERSEY
New Jersey Chapter, EFA
212 Durham Avenue, P.O. Box
  364
Metuchen, NJ 08840
(201) 548-4610

NEW MEXICO
Epilepsy Council of New Mexico
200 West First Street No. 742
Roswell, NM 88201
(505) 622-7065 or 623-9320

NEW YORK
Epilepsy Foundation of Nassau
  County
149 North Franklin Street
Hempstead, NY 11550
(516) 485-0977

NORTH CAROLINA
Epilepsy Association of North
  Carolina
1924 Vail Avenue
Charlotte, NC 28207
(704) 377-3619

NORTH DAKOTA
Epilepsy Foundation of North
  Dakota
319½ Fifth Street North, Suite B
Fargo, ND 58102
(701) 232-3371

OHIO
Epilepsy Association of Ohio
986 West Goodale Boulevard
Columbus, OH 43212
(614) 299-2195

OKLAHOMA
Oklahoma Foundation for Epilepsy
108 N.W. Twenty-fifth Street
Oklahoma City, OK 73103
(405) 528–1008

OREGON
Epilepsy Association of Oregon
718 West Burnside Street, Room
  204
Portland, OR 97209
(503) 228–7651

PENNSYLVANIA
Pennsylvania Division, EFA
P.O. Box 192
Lemoyne, PA 17043
(717) 561–0107

SOUTH CAROLINA
South Carolina Epilepsy
  Association
Medical University of South
  Carolina
P.O. Box 1159
Charleston, SC 29403
(803) 792–4513

SOUTH DAKOTA
Rehabilitation Center
405 South Third Street
Sioux Falls, SC 57105
(605) 339–6730

TENNESSEE
Memphis Epilepsy Foundation
1835 Union Avenue, Suite 209
Memphis, TN 38104
(901) 274–1720

TEXAS
Fort Worth/Tarrant County
  Epilepsy Association
3327 Winthrop Avenue No. 240
Forth Worth, TX 76116
(817) 731–4447

UTAH
Epilepsy Association of Utah
668 South 1300 East

Salt Lake City, UT 84102
(801) 583–4248

VERMONT
Epilepsy Association of Vermont
210 South Main Street
Rutland, VT 05701
(802) 775–1686

VIRGINIA
Epilepsy Association of Virginia
Suite 708, Medical Arts Building
Second and Franklin Streets
Richmond, VA 32319
(804) 644–0161

WASHINGTON
Epilepsy Association of King
  County
1016 First Avenue South
Seattle, WA 98134
(206) 447–9790

WEST VIRGINIA
Mountain State Epilepsy League
1319 Sixth Avenue
Huntington, WV 25701
(304) 525–6361 or 363–5008

WISCONSIN
Wisconsin Epilepsy Association
206 East Olin Avenue
Madison, WI 53703
(608) 255–9009

WYOMING
Wyoming Chapter, EFA
P.O. Box 9505
Casper, WY 82609
(307) 266–6336

GUAM
Epilepsy Foundation of Guam
P.O. Box 864
Agana, Guam 96910
(671) 477–8896 or 477–8897

PUERTO RICO
Sociedad Puertorriquenna de
  Ayuda Al Paciente con Epilepsia
  (Epilepsy Society of Puerto
  Rico)

Ruiz Soler
Calle Marginal-Final

Bayamon, PR 00619
(809) 782-6262

EPILEPSY ASSOCIATIONS OF CANADA

ALBERTA
Edmonton Epilepsy Association
308 Robert Armstrong Building
10012 Jasper Avenue
Edmonton, Alberta T5J 1R7,
Canada

Epilepsy Association of Calgary,
2422 Fifth Avenue N.W.
Calgary, Alberta T2N 0T2,
Canada

BRITISH COLUMBIA
Vancouver Neurological Center
1195 West Eighth Avenue
Vancouver, British Columbia V6H
1C5, Canada

British Columbia Epilepsy Society
1721 Richmond Road

Victoria, British Columbia V8R
1P7, Canada

ONTARIO
Epilepsy Association, Metro
Toronto
214 King Street West, Suite 214
Toronto, Ontario M5H 1K4,
Canada

Epilepsy Ontario
2160 Young Street
Toronto, Ontario M4S 2A9,
Canada

QUEBEC
Epilepsie-Montreal
493 Sherbrooke Street West
Montreal, Quebec H3A 1B6,
Canada

INTERNATIONAL ASSOCIATIONS FOR EPILEPSY

ASIA
The Japanese Epilepsy Association
4-20-19 Asagayakita
Suginami-ku
Tokyo, Japan

National Epilepsy Centre
c/o National Shizuoka-Higashi
Hospital
Higashi 886, Shizuoka 9MZ 420,
Japan

The Indian Epilepsy Association
251D, Naoroji Road
Bombay 400001, India

AUSTRALIA
West Australian Epilepsy
Association
14, Bagot Road

Subiaco, West Australia 6008

Epilepsy Association of South
Australia Inc.
Box 252 Post Office
Gleneig, South Australia 5045

Epilepsy Association of
Queensland
Room 511, Pennys Building
210 Queen Street
Brisbane, Queensland 4000

Epilepsy Association of Tasmania
P.O. Box 421
Sandy Bay, Tasmania 7005

CENTRAL AND SOUTH AMERICA
Asociación de Ligas contra la
Epilepsia de Chile

Casilla 4300
Valparaiso, Chile

Liga Colombiana contra la
Epilepsia
Apartado Aereo 2485
Cartagena, Colombia

Asociación de Lucha contra la
Epilepsia
Florida 165-7 piso-escr. 703
Buenos Aires, Argentina

EUROPE

Les Amis de la Ligue Nationale
Belge contre l'Epilepsie
135, Avenue Albert
Brussels 1060, Belgium

Dansk Epilepsiforening
Admiralgade 15
1066 Copenhagen K., Denmark

Irish Epilepsy Association
23, Dawson Street
Dublin 2, Ireland

British Epilepsy Association
Crowthorne House,
New Woklingham Road,
Wokingham, Berks. RG11 3 AY,
England

Sec. Epilepsialiitto Ry.
Kylakrikontie 23
00370 Helsinki 37, Finland

Hilfe für das Anfallskranke Kind,
23 Kiel, Hollanderey 5c. D. 2300
Kronshagen, West Germany

Greek National Association against
Epilepsy
45 Solonos Street
Athens, 135, Greece

Associazióne Lombarda per Lotta
contro l'Epilessia
Via Aurelio Saffi 9
Milan, Italy

B

RECOMMENDED READING
(BOOKS)

Many books and pamphlets have been written that deal with various handicaps, but few deal specifically and in nontechnical language with epilepsy. There are some references, however, which the authors of this book consider to be useful to adults with seizures and to parents of children with epilepsy or related neurological disorders. Some have been written for children. Wherever possible and when available, the address of the publisher and the purchase price are included.

BASIC READING — EPILEPSY

The Child with Convulsions: A Guide for Parents, Teachers, Counselors and Medical Personnel, by Henry Baird (1972). Grune and Stratton, 111 Fifth Avenue, New York, NY 10003. $7.50.

A well-organized book that covers the diagnosis and medical treatment of epilepsy for parents and professionals.

Epilepsy, by Alvin and Virginia Silverstein (1975). J. B. Lippincott, East Washington Square, Philadelphia, PA 19105. $6.95 hardcover, $1.95 paperback.

Intended for adolescents, this excellent book presents a description of epilepsy, the misconceptions, and treatment methods.

The Epilepsy Fact Book, by Harry Sands and Frances Minters (1977). F. A. Davis Co., 1915 Arch Street, Philadelphia, PA 19103. $5.50.

Presents basic facts about epilepsy, with a discussion of the problems and attitudes faced by persons with epilepsy. Includes a list of community services available to people with epilepsy.

The Epilepsy Form, by C. F. Hawkins and Harold Geist. Western Psychological Services, 12031 Wilshire Boulevard, Los Angeles, CA 90025. Package of 25 forms $6.60.

An eight-page booklet for recording and collecting the history, diagnosis, treatment, and rehabilitation data for persons with epilepsy. A time-saving method of bringing into structured form all information on and history of a patient for use by the parents as well as the entire clinic team.

Living with Chronic Neurological Disease: A Handbook for Patient and Family, by I. S. Cooper (1976). W. W. Norton and Co., 500 Fifth Avenue, New York, NY 10036. $4.95 paperback.

Describes the common neurological disorders, including epilepsy, in a readable manner.

Seizures, Epilepsy, and Your Child, by Jorge Lagos (1974). Harper and Row Pubs., 10 East Fifty-third Street, New York, NY 10022. $7.95.

A readable and practical book of questions and answers on epilepsy.

Understanding and Living with Brain Damage, by Patrick Logue (1975). Charles C Thomas, Publisher, 301–327 East Lawrence Street, Springfield, IL 62717. $8.50 hardcover, $5.95 paperback.

Discusses neurological conditions of aphasia, seizures, cerebral palsy, and minimal brain dysfunction, with emphasis on the individual and family.

BASIC READING — EDUCATION AND TRAINING AT HOME

Art and the Handicapped, by Zaidee Lindsay (1972). Van Nostrand Reinhold, 135 West Fiftieth Street, New York, NY 10020. $8.95 hardcover.

Presents many arts and crafts activities for the handicapped child.

Baby Learning through Baby Play, by Ira Gordon (1970), and

Child Learning through Child Play: Learning Activities for Two and Three-Year-Olds, by Ira Gordon et al. (1972). Both, St. Martin's Press, 175 Fifth Avenue, New York, NY 10010. $4.95 paperback (each).

These two books were not written specifically for the handicapped child, but they give a variety of games and activities that promote the development of a child and that would be appropriate for a child with seizure disorders.

Language Learning at Home, Council for Exceptional Children, 1920 Association Drive, Reston, VA 22091.

Teaching kits to be used at home, designed to strengthen motor, auditory, visual, and verbal development. Level I is for the three-to-five-year-old age group; Level II, for six to nine-year-olds. $35 per kit.

Living Fully: A Guide for Young People with a Handicap, by Sol Gordon (1975). John Day Co., Inc., 10 East Fifty-third Street, New York, NY 10022. $8.95 hardcover.

This book contains information for the professional and is also appropriate for adolescents and young adults and their families. It offers direct guidance and support for persons with handicaps toward attaining a satisfying and productive life.

Reading: An Auditory-Vocal Process, by Alexander Bannatyne (1973). Academic Therapy Pubs., Box 899, San Rafael, CA 94901. $3.00 paperback.

A short, comprehensive book that covers the language basics of reading, including phonetics, articulation, auditory discrimination, and memory. The book explains the complex processes in reading.

See What I Can Do! by Maya Doray (1973). Prentice-Hall, Inc., Englewood Cliffs, NJ 07632. $4.95.

A book the child can use on his own to stimulate physical development of muscles and motor coordination.

Speech and Language Delay, by Ray Battin and Olaf Haug (1973). Charles C. Thomas, Publisher, 301–327 East Lawrence Street, Springfield, IL 62717. $5.50.

A basic handbook on speech and language delay, providing parents with information on the process of language development and a structured plan for parents to follow to improve their child's speech.

Steps to Independence: A Skills Training Series for Children with Special Needs, Research Press, P.O. Box 317750, Champaign, IL 61820.

Booklets for parents to teach self-help and independent living skills. $7.95 each.

TA for Teens (and Other Important People), by Alvyn Freed (1976). Jalmar Press, address above. $7.95 paperback.

A book for teenagers to help them understand their feelings and develop a closer and more satisfying relationship with their parents, teachers, and friends. Offers options and positive suggestions for growth.

TA for Tots (and Other Prinzes), by Alvyn Freed (1973). Jalmar Press, 6501 Elvas Avenue, Sacramento, CA 95819. $5.95 paperback.

A unique book designed to help children and adolescents understand their feelings and learn about behavior. It is a primer to Transactional Analysis (TA) easily understood by children.

Teach Your Child to Talk: A Parent's Guide, by David Pushaw (1976). Dantree Press, Inc., 44 West Sixty-second Street, New York, NY 10023. $5.95 paperback.

Presents typical speech and language development patterns by age, from birth to age five. Includes helpful sections on early identification of language problems along with suggestions for helping the child with delayed speech development.

They Too Can Succeed: A Practical Guide for Learning Disabled Children, edited by Doreen Kronik (1969). Academic Therapy Pubs., Box 899, San Rafael, CA 94901. $3.75 paperback.

A collection of articles helpful to achieving success in the role of parent of a child with special learning needs.

Toys and Games for Educationally Handicapped Children, by Charlotte Buist and

Jerome Schulman (1976). Charles C. Thomas, Publisher, 301–327 East Lawrence Street, Springfield, IL 62717. $9.50 hardcover.

An extensive catalogue of toys and games appropriate to different age levels and educational disabilities in such areas as fine- and gross-motor skills, visual and auditory perception, conceptualization, and verbal expression.

The Tuned-In, Turned-On Book about Learning Problems, by Marnell Hayes (1974). Academic Therapy Pubs., Box 899, San Rafael, CA 94901. $2.50 paperback; $7.95 for 90-minute cassette tape of book.

This book is appropriate for pre-adolescent and adolescent youths with learning problems. Presents direct, factual information, written in a style for this age. A unique feature is the cassette tape to assist those who have difficulty reading.

What About Me? The LD Adolescent, by Doreen Kronik et al. (1975). Academic Therapy Pubs., Box 899, San Rafael, CA 94901. $6.50 paperback.

Presents a comprehensive overview of learning disabled adolescent problems, including education, family relationships, and methods of fostering positive emotional growth. Not oriented specifically to seizure disorders, but helpful for learning problems often associated with epilepsy.

BASIC READING — CHILD MANAGEMENT

Behavior Guides, by Howard Sloan, Jr. Research Press, P.O. Box 3177, Champaign, IL 61820. $1.25 each, paperback; $6.25 complete set.

Five short manuals with step-by-step activities to change specific behaviors, written in simple, understandable language. (Titles are *Stop That Fighting; Dinner's Ready; Not Till Your Room's Clean; No More Whining; Because I Said So.*)

The First Twelve Months of Life. 1971 edition, Grosset and Dunlap, Inc., 51 Madison Avenue, New York, NY 10010, $9.95 hardcover. 1978 Bantam Book (paperback), carried in bookstores, $2.75.

An excellent description of the development of a child during the important first year. Fully detailed monthly growth charts of the sequence of motor, language, and social areas. Presents what parents need to watch for, and how they might assist. Can be used by parents of older children with developmental disabilities.

The Hyperactive Child: A Handbook for Parents, by Paul Wender (1973). Crown Pubs., 1 Park Avenue South, New York, NY 10016. $3.95 paperback.

A good description of hyperactivity in contrast to normal child activity. Discusses causes and methods of treatment.

Little People: Guidelines for Common Sense Child Rearing, by Edward Christopherson (1977). H & H Enterprises, Inc., P.O. Box 1070, Lawrence, KS 66044. $8.50 hardcover.

254 / RECOMMENDED READING

This is a helpful little book based on the premise that parents should pay greater attention to the child's desirable behavior than to other forms. It provides comprehensive guidelines for child development, discipline, and specific problems of behavior, and advice for seeking and working with professionals in helping the child.

Living with Children: New Methods for Parents and Teachers, by Gerald Patterson and Elizabeth Gullion (1968; 7th printing 1974). Research Press, Box 3177, Champaign, IL 61820. $3.95 paperback.

Of all the books available on behavior modification, this little book remains one of the best in the field for parents. It is practical, easy to understand, and organized in a programmed (self-learning) format.

The Retarded Child: Answers to Questions Parents Ask, by A. Attwell and D. Clabby (1972). Western Psychological Services, 12031 Wilshire Boulevard, Los Angeles, CA 90025. $5.95 paperback.

A basic information manual on mental retardation, with answers to the questions most frequently asked by parents. Useful for parents and professionals.

What Every Child Would Like His Parents to Know, by Lee Salk (1972). Warner Books, 75 Rockefeller Plaza, New York, NY 10019. $1.95 paperback, carried by bookstores.

A well-written, readable book covering a variety of topics, but especially useful in the areas of discipline, death, sex education, and for helping the child through emotional troubles.

NONFICTION — EPILEPSY AND RELATED DISORDERS

Be Not Afraid, by Robin White (1972). Berkley Pubs., 200 Madison Avenue, New York, NY 10016. $1.25 paperback.

A sensitive and well-written book by the father of a child with epilepsy, strongly recommended to parents. Describes the strains — emotional, financial, physical — involved in dealing with severe epilepsy.

A Difference in the Family, by Helen Featherstone (1980). Basic Books, 10 East Fifty-third Street, New York, NY 10022. $13.95.

A sensitive discussion, by the mother of a profoundly brain-damaged child, about the impact of such a handicap upon relationships with family, friends, and professionals.

He's My Brother, by Joe Lasker (1972). Whitman and Co., 560 West Lake Street, Chicago, IL 60606. $3.95 paperback.

A story about a boy with a learning disability, written by his older brother. Not designed specifically for seizure problems, but presents the handicap sensitively and is recommended for developing awareness of subtle handicaps in young children.

How to Live with Epilepsy, by Carroll Lunt (1961). Twayne Pubs., 70 Lincoln Street, Boston, MA 02111.

A very readable book based upon the author's experiences with her son's epilepsy.

Me Too, by Vera and Bill Cleaver (1973). J. B. Lippincott, East Washington Square, Philadelphia, PA 19105. $6.95 hardcover.

A good book for developing awareness of and empathy with the handicapped child. A sensitive, well-written story about a twelve-year-old retarded twin. This book is appropriate for pre-adolescents and for adolescent siblings of a handicapped child.

No Time for Tears, by Katheryn Patterson (1965). Johnson Pubs., 820 South Michigan Avenue, Chicago, IL 60605. $3.95.

The author tells about her ill health, her epilepsy, and her becoming the mother of a hydrocephalic child and learning to cope.

"Patty Wilson's Magnificent Marathon," by Sheila Cragg. *Reader's Digest*, April 1978.

Run, Patty, Run, bySheila Cragg. Harper and Row Pubs., 10 East Fifty-third Street, New York, NY 10022.

Tony Coelho: "Congressman Makes His Own Epilepsy a Campaign Issue to Break the Old Taboos," interview by C. Crawford-Mason. *People* 16 (August 17, 1981).

FICTION, WITH EPILEPSY AS ALL OR PART OF THE THEME

The Idiot, by Fedor Dostoevsky. Available in paperback, at most bookstands.

A novel, based on the author's life, about a person subject to seizures who had been institutionalized for part of his life.

Nobody's Brother, by C. F. Griffin (1960). Barrie & Rockliff, Pubs., London.

Portrays an adolescent with epilepsy and his life in the slums of New York.

Seizure, by Charles Mee (1978). M. Evans and Co., 216 East Forty-ninth Street, New York, NY 10017. $8.95 hardcover.

A dramatized portrayal of the feelings and experiences of a surgeon and his patient in the diagnosis and surgery of a brain tumor.

Why Have the Birds Stopped Singing? by Zoa Sherburne (1974). William Morrow and Co., 105 Madison Avenue, New York, NY 10016. $4.95 paperback.

A well-written Gothic novel about a girl with epilepsy who was transported back in time and mistreated because of having epilepsy. Most suitable for adolescent girls.

BASIC READING — MISCELLANEOUS

The Disabled and Their Parents: A Counseling Challenge, edited by Leo Buscaglia (1975). Charles B. Slack, Inc., 6900 Grove Road, Thorofare, NJ 08086. $8.95 hardcover.

An excellent collection of chapters written by both professional and lay contributors and edited by a leader in special education.

The Exceptional Parent, P.O. Box 4944, Manchester, NH 03108. A magazine for parents of handicapped children ($14 per year).

A Primer on Due Process: Education Decisions for Handicapped Children, by Alan Abelson, Nancy Bolick, and Jayne Hass (1975). Council for Exceptional Children, 1920 Association Drive, Reston, VA 22091. $4.95 paperback. This is a good handbook regarding "due process" procedures to safeguard the rights of children in the educational system. It covers placement and management in special classes.

TECHNICAL READING — EPILEPSY

Advances in Epileptology: Proceedings, Epilepsy International Symposium (tenth), edited by Juhn Wade, M.D., and J. Kiffin Penry, M.D. (1980). Raven Press Pubs., 1140 Avenue of the Americas, New York, NY 10036; see in particular "A Collaborative Study of the Teratogenicity and Fetal Toxicity of Antiepileptic Drugs in Japan," by T. Okuma, R. Takabashi, T. Wada, Y. Sato, and Y. Nakane (pp. 511–517).

Complex Partial Seizures and Their Treatment, Advances in Neurology vol. II, edited by J. Kiffin Penry, M.D., and David D. Daley, M.D. (1975). Raven Press Pubs., address above; see in particular "Hematologic Toxicity of Carbamazepine," by A. V. Pisciotta (pp. 355–368).

Comprehensive Management of Epilepsy in Infancy, Childhood and Adolescence, by Samuel Livingston (1972). Charles C. Thomas, Publisher, 301–327 East Lawrence Avenue, Springfield, IL 62717.

Epilepsy: A Clinical and Social Analysis of 1,020 Adults with Epileptic Seizures, by Palle Juul-Jensen (1963). Munksgaard, Copenhagen, Denmark.

Epilepsy: The Eighth International Symposium, edited by J. Kiffin Penry, M.D. (1977). Raven Press Pubs., 1140 Avenue of the Americas, New York, NY 10036.

Epilepsy Rehabilitation, Epilepsy Foundation of America, edited by George N. Wright (1975). Little, Brown and Co., 34 Beacon Street, Boston, MA 02106.

Epileptic Seizures: Clinical and Electrographic Features, Diagnosis and Treatment, by Henri Gastaut, M.D., and Roger Broughton, M.D. (1972). Charles C. Thomas, Publisher, 301–327 East Lawrence Avenue, Springfield, IL 62717.

"Isolated Flying Spot Detection of Radiodensity Discontinuities — Displaying the Internal Structure Pattern of a Complex Object," by William H. Oldendorf, M.D. *IRE Transactions on Bio-Medical Electronics* 8 (1961): 68–72.

Plan for Nationwide Action on Epilepsy, Report of the Commission for the Control of Epilepsy and Its Consequences, vols. I–IV, by Richard

Masland et al. (1977). U.S. Government Printing Office, Washington, DC, Dept. of Health and Human Services Publication 78–276.

The Prognosis of Patients with Epilepsy, by E. Rodin, M.D. (1968). Charles C Thomas, Publisher, 301–327 East Lawrence Avenue, Springfield, IL 62717.

"Remission of Seizures and Relapse in Patients with Epilepsy," by J. Annegers, W. Hauser, and L. Elvebock. *Epilepsia* 20 (1979): 729–737.

A Textbook of Epilepsy, by John Laidlaw and Alan Richans (1976). Churchill Livingstone Publishers, through Medical Division of Longman, Inc., 19 West Forty-fourth Street, New York, NY 10036.

C

FREE OR LOW-COST
PAMPHLETS

The following pamphlets are available through the Epilepsy Foundation of America, 4351 Garden City Drive, Landover, MD 20785. Single copies of EFA brochures are free.

Answers to the Most Frequent Questions People Ask about Epilepsy (1977). 20¢.
Are You As Informed As You Think You Are? 10¢.
Because You Are My Friend (1979). 10¢. Excellent for the pre-adolescent to read on his own, or for a person to read to a younger child. Explains epilepsy in a child's language, provides an opportunity for dialogue, discusses types of seizures, medication, prejudices, etc. A simple yet sensitive child's introduction to epilepsy. Also available in Spanish.
Benjamin (1972). Available from the Epilepsy Society of Massachusetts, 20 Providence Street, Suite 601–603, Boston, MA 02116. Cartoon coloring booklet. Used with children in class in preparing the Epilepsy School Alert program; can also be used with an individual child to understand epilepsy in a peer.
Employment Action on Epilepsy: A Guide for Employers and Employees (1978).
Epilepsy and Insurance (1978).
Epilepsy School Alert Kit. $4.00.
Epilepsy: The Teacher's Role (1971). 10¢.
Epilepsy: You and Your Child (1979). 40¢.
Facts and Figures on the Epilepsies and Other Neurological Dysfunctions (1976). 10¢.
Medications for Epilepsy (1979). Price to be established.
A Patient's Guide to EEG. 4¢.
Recognition of First Aid for Those with Epilepsy: Guidelines for Those Who Meet the Public (1973). 10¢.

Research into the Epilepsies (1975).
The Role of the School Nurse in the Understanding and Treatment of Epilepsy (1974). 10¢.
Seizure Man: First Aid for Seizures (comic-book format; 1980).
Teacher's Tips about the Epilepsies (1973). 6¢.
To What Extent and in What Ways Can Epilepsy and Its Consequences Be Prevented? (1978). 10¢.
What Everyone Should Know About Epilepsy (1978). 10¢.
Workman's Compensation and Epilepsy (1972).
First Aid for Epilepsy Wallet Card (1980). 10¢.
Medication Record. 10¢.
Parents' Information Kit (1980). $1.00.

The following pamphlets are available through the U.S. Government Printing Office, Washington, DC 20402:
Child with Epilepsy (35). 10¢.
Epilepsia — Esperanza en la Investigación. 35¢.
Learning to Talk: Speech, Hearing, and Language Problems in the Pre-School Child. 45¢.
National Park Guide for the Handicapped. 40¢.
Your Child from 1 to 6 (30). 20¢.
Your Child from 6 to 12 (324). 25¢.

MISCELLANEOUS PAMPHLETS AND SOURCES

The Dental Implications of Epilepsy (1977). Department of Health and Human Services Publication 79–5217, Public Health Service, Rockville, MD 20857. Single copy free.

Epilepsy and the School Age Child. Comprehensive Epilepsy Program, 2829 University Avenue S.E., Suite 608, Minneapolis, MN 55414. Single copy free.

Facts About: The Mental Health of Children. U.S. Department of Health and Human Services, 5600 Fishers Lane, Rockville, MD 20852. Single copy free.

Genetic Counseling in Family Planning. National Association for Retarded Citizens, 381 Elliot Street, Newton Upper Falls, MA 02164. Single copy free.

Handbook for Parents, by H. Barrows and E. Goldensohn. Ayerst Laboratories, 685 Third Avenue, New York, NY 10017. Single copy free.

Hope through Research: Epilepsy and *Hope through Research: Learning Disabilities due to Minimal Brain Dysfunction.* Both available through U.S. Department of Health and Human Services, National Institute of Neurological and Communicative Disorders and Stroke, Building 31, 9000 Rockville Pike, Bethesda, MD 20205. Single copy free.

Infant Stimulation: A Pamphlet for Parents of Multiple-Handicapped Children, by Sandra Hoffman. University of Kansas Medical Center, Children's Rehabilitation Unit, Rainbow Boulevard at Thirty-ninth Street, Kansas City, KS 66103. Single copy free.

Questions and Answers on Birth Defects. March of Dimes, 250 West Fifty-seventh Street, New York, NY 10019. Single copy free.

A Speech Pathologist Talks to the Parents of a Nonverbal Child, by Harriet Dunbar (1969). National Easter Seal Society, 2023 West Ogden Avenue, Chicago, IL 60612. Single copy free.

Thoughts on Parenting the Child with Epilepsy, by Elizabeth Bauer. Comprehensive Epilepsy Program, 2829 University Avenue, S.E., Suite 608, Minneapolis, MN 55414. Single copy free.

You and Your Seizures (1978). For children ages seven through thirteen. Epilepsy Foundation of North Carolina, Inc., 1924 Vail Avenue, Charlotte, NC 28207. Single copy free.

D

FILMS ON EPILEPSY

The following films and audiovisual materials are available for use with a variety of audiences. We have included what we consider to be the best materials available at this time. The sources are noted for those not obtainable from the EFA. All others may be ordered for loan or purchase from Epilepsy Materials Center, Epilepsy Foundation of America, 4351 Garden City Drive, Landover, MD 20785.

A service charge of $6 covers the shipping, handling, and insurance on the loan films. Payment must accompany the order. Make checks payable to the Epilepsy Foundation of America. The charge allows for showing the film for three consecutive days. Additional charges will be levied for films held longer. The Centers suggest ordering the film(s) at least six to eight weeks in advance. Indicate the showing date preference and some alternative later dates.

Antiepileptic Medications - Why? (slide/audio cassette materials, color, produced by Comprehensive Epilepsy Program, University of Minnesota). Designed as a patient education package to explain anticonvulsant medications, therapeutic range, and the need for compliance. Suitable for adolescents and adults.

Because You Are My Friend (slide-tape presentation, color, 5 mins., produced by EFA). Based on the EFA pamphlet of the same name, this unit is attractive and colorful, with the narration in a child's voice. Designed to be used in conjunction with the Epilepsy School Alert program for young children (ages six to twelve) to help understand a child with epilepsy. Available for use from most local EFA affiliate chapters. It may also be purchased for $25 from the EFA Materials Center.

Benjamin (16mm, color, 5 mins., produced by the Epilepsy Society of Massachusetts, 20 Providence Street, Suite 601–603, Boston, Massachusetts 02116). Animated cartoon film designed to explain epilepsy to young children (ages five through nine).

Build Your Own City — Build Your Own Walls - A Person with Epilepsy (16 mm, color, 28 mins., produced by Abbott Laboratories). A new film narrated by television star Michael Learned, featuring the discovery of epilepsy in a young man. Recommended for general audiences.

Doctors Talk about Epilepsy (16mm, color, 24 mins., produced by EFA). This is an excellent film intended primarily for physicians, but also suitable for other health professionals or persons already knowledgeable about epilepsy. It features the International Classification of Epilepsies and describes anticonvulsant treatment.

Epilepsy: Don't Look Away (16mm, color, 10 mins., produced by EFA). A film to show to the general public for a lay understanding of epilepsy and how to help with the problems associated with the disorder.

Epilepsy: First Aid for Seizures (16 mm, color, 12 mins., produced by Comprehensive Epilepsy Program, University of Minnesota). This new film demonstrates the first aid necessary for absence, generalized tonic-clonic, and complex partial seizures, as well as appropriate precautions for school and employment. Suitable for adolescents and adults.

Epilepsy: For Those Who Teach (16mm, color, 13 mins., produced by EFA). A film designed to help teachers understand epilepsy and how to handle seizures in the classroom. It illustrates how to give needed emotional support to the child with epilepsy.

Epilepsy Is . . . (slide-audio cassette or filmstrip-audio cassette materials, color, 10–15 mins., produced by Comprehensive Epilepsy Program, University of Minnesota). This new material is designed to teach what happens during a seizure and what aid to provide. The material is available as Program I, designed for children ages five to twelve; and Program II, designed for adolescents twelve years and above and for adults. Specify filmstrip or slide. The audio tapes are available with either audible tone or synchronized equipment. The material may be purchased from the EFA Materials Center.

Epilepsy: Pass the Word (16mm, color, 12 mins., produced by EFA). Designed for employers, managers, and unions, to present a practical view of epilepsy and employment.

I'm the Same as Everyone Else (16mm, color, 26 mins., produced by and available from the Epilepsy Association of Metro Toronto, 214 King Street, Suite 214, Toronto, Ontario M5H 1K4). An appealing film for adolescents, concentrating on the candid conversations, activities, and emotions of young persons with epilepsy. Suitable for adolescents and adults.

Images of Epilepsy (16mm, color, 18 mins., produced by the Colorado

Epilepsy Association, 1835 Gaylord Street, Denver, CO 80206). An excellent film to create awareness and understanding of epilepsy through unique presentations of petit mal, focal and grand mal seizures. Suitable for children ages ten and older and adults.

Let's Talk It Over (16mm, color, 6 mins., produced by and available from the Encyclopaedia Britannica Educational Corp., 1822 Pickwick Avenue, Glenview, IL 60025, or 2494 Teagarden Street, San Leandro, CA 94577). This animated cartoon film tells the story of a child with absence seizures who fails to respond during a kickball game, and how the other children learn about his epilepsy. The film is designed to promote awareness in young children (ages five through twelve).

Modern Concepts of Epilepsy (16mm, color, 20 mins., produced by EFA). A good film for professional groups, such as nurses or counselors, that shows the types of seizures.

Nurses Talk about Epilepsy (16mm, color, 13 mins., produced by EFA). This film covers the nurse's role in handling persons with epilepsy and drug therapy. Appropriate for nurses and the general public.

Many of these films are also available on free loan from the Comprehensive Epilepsy Programs. Contact the CEP in your area for a list. Other films are available for special audiences. Contact the EFA for lists.

GLOSSARY OF TERMS

ABLATE: To remove, for example, by surgery.

ABSENCE SEIZURE: A seizure characterized by momentary lapse of consciousness; petit mal.

ACETAZOLAMIDE (Diamox): A second-line drug generally used as an adjunct to other drugs, especially in female patients whose seizures are most often associated with the menstrual period.

ACETYLCHOLINE: An ester of choline normally present in the body that has the role of transmission of an impulse from one nerve fiber to another.

ACTH (corticotropin): A hormone secreted by the anterior pituitary gland, the function of which is to stimulate production of certain chemical compounds in the adrenal cortex.

ACTING OUT: An expression of emotional conflict (usually subconscious), or of strong feelings of hostility (or of love). The person is usually unaware of the relationship between the actions and his conflicts or feelings.

ACTIVE EPILEPSY: Seizures not under control for a period of five years without medication.

ADAPTIVE BEHAVIOR: An autocorrective (subconscious) means by which one adjusts to his environment.

ADVERSIVE SEIZURE: A form of focal seizure in which the eyes, head, or trunk often deviate to one side. One arm may remain raised during the attack.

ADVOCACY: Support, as for a cause.

AFEBRILE: Without any evidence of fever.

AFFECT: The feeling experienced in connection with an emotion.

AFFECTIVE SEIZURE: A seizure, usually focal or temporal lobe, accompanied by emotional reactions (laughing, crying, etc.).

AGNOSIA: An organic brain disorder resulting in the inability to recognize and interpret sensory impressions.

AKINETIC SEIZURE: A generalized seizure, usually in children, with loss of muscle control and of widely varying duration, often characterized by falling or loss of consciousness.

ALKALOSIS: Increased alkalinity of the blood.

ALPHA RHYTHM: An electrical rhythm of about 10 oscillations per second, characteristic of the brain during normal wakefulness.

AMENTIA: Mental retardation, usually organic, due to developmental lack of brain tissue.

AMINO ACIDS: Organic compounds, essential components of the protein molecule.

ANALEPTIC: A substance that has a stimulatory or convulsive-producing agent.

ANALGESIA: A condition in which the sense of pain is minimized or stopped.

ANEURYSM: A sac filled with blood, formed by pressure on a weakened artery, vein, or the heart.

ANOMALIES, CRANIAL: Structural abnormalities of the skull.

ANOMALY: Abnormality.

ANOXIA: A condition caused by lack of oxygen in the blood, rendering tissue functioning inadequate. Cerebral anoxia, often a factor in mental retardation, is a lack of oxygen in the brain during the birth process.

ANTIBODY: A substance produced in the blood as a reaction against foreign substances introduced in the bloodstream.

ANTICONVULSANT: Any agent (drug) used to control seizures.

ANTIEPILEPTIC: An anticonvulsant used to treat epilepsy in humans. Only a few anticonvulsants are actually considered as antiepileptics.

ANXIETY: A generalized feeling of worry or apprehension without apparent cause.

APATHY: A feeling of indifference in which the person loses interest in himself.

APHASIA: A loss of ability to pronounce words or to name common objects. Motor aphasia victims may retain the understanding of words but lose the memory traces necessary to produce the sounds. It may also involve written expression. Sensory aphasia involves the loss of ability to comprehend the meaning of words or phrases. The patient will usually have a mixed type of expressive and receptive aphasia.

APNEA: Temporary cessation of respiration, caused by an excess of oxygen in the blood.

APRAXIA: A condition caused by lesions in the cerebral cortex, resulting in an inability to perform certain physical movements.

ARRHYTHMIA: Irregularity, as cardiac arrhythmia (heart-rhythm).

ARTERIOGRAM: An X ray of an artery after the injection of an opaque substance for clarity. In the diagnosis of epilepsy, it refers to X ray of arteries in the brain.

ARTICULATION: The movement of the muscles used in forming speech sounds.

ASYMPTOMATIC: Showing no symptoms.

ATAXIA: Loss of muscular coordination; a form of cerebral palsy involving abnormal muscular coordination.

ATHETOSIS: A condition in which organic brain injury (for example, cerebral palsy) causes continual, slow changes of position of the extremities.

ATONIC: Referring to loss of muscle tone.

ATONIC SEIZURE: A generalized seizure, involving a sagging of the head, body, or limbs. Atonic seizures are usually brief.

ATROPHY: A wasting or reduction in size of a structure by disease, disuse, or injury.

ATTACK: A seizure or episode in which there is a clinical change in one's state, with a change in the normal symptoms.

ATTENTION: The process of focusing perception on a single object or event.

AUDIOLOGIST: A specialist in the field of hearing.

AUDIOMETRY: The measurement of hearing.

AUDITORY: Pertaining to the sense of hearing.

AURA: Sensory, motor, autonomic, or "feeling" sensations recognized by a person with epilepsy as preceding a seizure. It is actually the seizure discharge starting in a certain area of brain tissue.

AUTISM: Usually associated with children, and considered related to schizophrenia, this condition manifests itself in extreme withdrawal, stimulus reaction failure, and inappropriate verbal and gestural behavior. Prognosis is usually considered poor.

AUTONOMIC MANIFESTATIONS: Sensory or motor manifestations that often occur in connection with generalized seizures. They sometimes occur as an aura, and may involve vomiting, perspiration, hypertension, lack of bowel control, etc.

AUTONOMIC NERVOUS SYSTEM: The part of the nervous system not ordinarily subject to voluntary control.

AVMS: Arteriovenous malformations.

BAYLEY SCALES OF INFANT DEVELOPMENT: A test used to measure the developmental progress of infants and young children to age thirty months.

BEHAVIOR MODIFICATION: A technique of changing (modifying) behavior through reinforcement of desirable behavior by token rewards, toward the concept that the desirable behavior eventually becomes its own reinforcement.

BENDER-GESTALT TEST: A test in which the person is asked to copy nine simple designs from printed cards. Drawings may suggest perceptual, psychological, or neurological disorder as interpreted by experienced examiners.

BILIRUBIN: A reddish yellow bile pigment in the blood, which can cause brain damage through decreased oxygen uptake.

BIOFEEDBACK: The process of providing evidence to a person of the states of his body functions in order that he may learn to exert control over specific functions.

BLINDNESS: Legal blindness is defined as 20/200 (or worse) vision in the better eye after correction. Vision of 20/70 in the better eye after correction would be termed partial sight.

BLOCKING: Interruption in thought, memory, or speech, usually due to subconscious emotional factors, but which could also be organic.

BLOOD-LEVEL MONITORING: Determining by laboratory tests the level of medication in the bloodstream, as a guide for effectiveness and/or needed change in medication.

BONE AGE: A means of measuring and predicting growth in terms of bone development.

BRAIN POTENTIALS: Tiny rhythmic electrical discharges given off by the cerebral cortex and measured by the EEG.

BRAIN SCAN: An X ray of the brain.

BRAINSTEM: A group of brain structures, including the pons, medulla, and cerebellum.

BRAIN WAVE: The recording of electrical activity of the brain.

CARBAMAZEPINE (Tegretol): An anticonvulsant for control of focal-onset, secondarily generalized seizures, such as psychomotor or temporal lobe, and secondarily generalized tonic-clonic seizures, as well as generalized tonic-clonic seizures.

CATAPLEXY: A sudden, brief attack usually evoked by a sudden or unexpected emotional stimulation and characterized by loss of muscle strength. Cataplexy is not associated with any seizure discharge in the brain, but does occur in a disorder called narcolepsy.

CATHARSIS: A therapeutic release through talking or understanding of conscious material, accompanied by the appropriate emotional reaction.

CAT SCAN: Computerized axial tomography. A new technique of taking X-ray pictures of the brain and putting the information through a computer, which will print out all the densities on a certain plane.

CATTELL INFANT INTELLIGENCE SCALE: A test for measuring intellectual and physical development in infants from two months to thirty months old.

CELONTIN. *See* Methsuximide.

CENTRAL NERVOUS SYSTEM (CNS): The spinal cord and the brain.

CEPHALIC DELIVERY: The normal (head-first) position of the fetus during delivery.

CEREBELLAR ATAXIA: Muscular incoordination resulting from injury to the cerebellum.

CEREBELLUM: The part of the brain involved with muscle coordination and the maintenance of body equilibrium.

CEREBRAL ANOXIA: Lack of oxygen in the brain during the birth process.

CEREBRAL CORTEX: The outer surface layer of the brain.

CEREBRAL HEMISPHERE: Either lateral half of the brain.

CEREBRAL LESION: Any type of pathological abnormality of the brain.

CEREBRAL PALSY: A nonprogressive disorder caused by an injury to the brain at birth or in early infancy, causing permanent motor impairment.

CEREBROSPINAL FLUID: A clear fluid contained within the brain cavities and spinal cord.

CEREBRUM: The largest part of the brain, located in the upper region of the cranium.

CETA: The Comprehensive Employment and Training Act, a federally funded program to prepare low-income or handicapped persons for employment.

CHOREA: A widespread jerking or twitching of muscles.

CHOREIFORM: Of the nature of chorea.

CHROMOSOMES: The carriers of the genes within the nucleus of the cell.

CHRONIC: Persisting over a long period of time.

CHRONOLOGICAL AGE (CA): Actual life age expressed in terms of years and/or months.

CLEFT PALATE: A congenital failure in the development of the roof of the mouth.

CLIMATE: Psychological atmosphere or feeling tone present in a classroom or group, determined by the individual attitudes within the group.

CLINICAL: Referring to the professional observation and treatment of patients.

CLONAZEPAM (Clonopin): An anticonvulsant drug used for control of absence or myoclonic seizures.

CLONIC SEIZURE: A generalized spasm or seizure in infants, characterized by alternating rigidity and relaxation of muscles. Seizures may last longer than one minute and are associated with loss of consciousness and autonomic manifestations.

CLONOPIN. See Clonazepam.

COGNITIVE: Referring to mental processes such as comprehension, judgment, reasoning, etc.

COMPLEX PARTIAL SEIZURES: Seizures arising from the temporal lobe (psychomotor), which are partial in nature and are usually accompanied by strange, subjective feelings such as illusions, visions, strangeness or familiarity, or involuntary movements. Usually not remembered by the person.

COMPREHENSIVE MENTAL HEALTH CENTERS: Funded centers

providing free or low-cost mental health services to persons within certain geographically defined areas.

COMPUTERIZED AXIAL TOMOGRAPHY. *See* CAT scan.

CONDITIONING: A learning process in which behavior becomes attached to a new stimulus.

CONGENITAL: Refers to conditions present at birth, but acquired during the fetal development; not inherited.

CONGENITAL MALFORMATION: A defect existing in a child at the time of birth and due to some influence during pregnancy.

CONVULSION: A violent, involuntary series of muscular contractions (seizure).

CONVULSIVE THRESHOLD: The level above which convulsions occur.

CORPUS CALLOSUM: A large nerve tract connecting the right and left hemisphere of the cerebrum, allowing coordination of and cooperation in the functions of each hemisphere.

CORTICAL EXCISION: Surgical removal of a part of the cortex of the brain.

CORTICAL SEIZURE: A partial (focal) seizure caused by excessive discharge in one portion of the cerebral cortex. These seizures, though focal, are often known to spread and to become generalized.

CORTICOTROPIN. *See* ACTH.

CRANIAL NERVES: The twelve sensory and motor nerves that connect directly with the brain.

CRETINISM: An abnormal condition, usually congenital, caused by lack of thyroid secretion, and characterized by stunted physical and mental development.

CRYPTOGENIC EPILEPSY: Term applied to those acquired forms of epilepsy whose cause is unknown (idiopathic).

CULTURAL DEPRIVATION (cultural disadvantage): Reduction or lack of environmental stimulation (social, economical, educational, cultural, etc.).

DD: Developmentally Disabled. *See* Developmental Disability.

DEAFNESS: Legal deafness is a hearing loss in the better ear after correction of 70 decibels or more, or a loss of 50 decibels or more sustained in early childhood. A loss of from 45 to 70 decibels would be termed "severely hard of hearing" (or loss of 30 decibels sustained in early childhood).

DEMENTIA: Formerly used to designate psychosis; now refers to intellectual loss due to organic causes. Is sometimes associated with cerebral pathology which causes epilepsy.

DENTITION: The forming and development of teeth.

DENVER DEVELOPMENTAL SCREENING TEST: A test for attaining an estimate of the development and behavior in an infant or child up to six years old.

DEPAKENE: *See* Valproic acid.

DEPRESSION: Morbid dejection or melancholy, varying in intensity from neurosis to psychosis.

DEVELOPMENTAL CENTERS FOR THE HANDICAPPED (DCH): State-supported educational centers for severely handicapped persons ages three to twenty-one for whom no other school program is available.

DEVELOPMENTAL DISABILITY: A disability due to mental retardation, cerebral palsy, autism, epilepsy, or a neurological condition that originated in childhood, is likely to continue, and is a substantial handicap to the individual.

DEVELOPMENTAL TASKS: Those functions that follow a developmental sequence, the successful completion of one leading to another.

DEXTROAMPHETAMINE (Dexedrine): A drug used to counteract drowsiness resulting from a more sedating medication; a mild anticonvulsant in its own right.

DIAGNOSIS: The procedure by which the nature of a disease or condition is determined.

DIAMOX. *See* Acetazolamide.

DIAZEPAM (Valium): A minor tranquilizer, also used as a skeletal muscle relaxant and as an adjunct for controlling myoclonic and atonic seizures.

DIENCEPHALIC EPILEPSY. *See* Autonomic manifestations.

DILANTIN. *See* Phenytoin.

DISINHIBITION: Random, uncontrolled behavior, often associated with emotional or neurological involvement.

DISSOCIATION: A defense process that operates automatically (subconsciously), in which significance and affect are separated from an idea or situation. Includes hysterical reactions (such as amnesia, functional paralysis, etc.).

DIURNAL SEIZURE: A seizure occurring during the day (when the person is awake), as opposed to a nocturnal seizure.

DRUG GENERIC NAME: Name based on the chemical composition of the drug.

DRUG INTOXICATION: Drug poisoning because of the toxic effects of the drug on a person.

DRUG TOLERANCE: Reduced effectiveness of a particular drug, usually after continued use. Either a greater dosage or another drug is usually indicated.

DRUG TOXICITY. *See* Drug intoxication.

DRUG TRADE NAME: Name used by a company to market a drug. Common name of drug.

DYSARTHRIA: Impairment of speech due to organic disorders of the nervous system.

DYSGRAPHIA: A neurological disorder resulting in writing difficulties.

DYSLALIA: Impairment of speech caused by damage to the speech organs rather than to the nervous system.

DYSLEXIA: An inability to deal with printed symbols; impaired ability to read.

DYSPHASIA: Impairment of speech resulting from a brain lesion.

DYSPHORIA: Emotional state of anxiety or depression, as opposed to euphoria.

DYSRHYTHMIA, CEREBRAL: Disturbance or irregularity in the electrical impulses of the brain, as recorded on the EEG.

ECHOLALIA: An automatic repetition of words or phrases spoken by others, frequently found in connection with certain schizophrenic disorders.

EDUCATION OF ALL HANDICAPPED CHILDREN ACT: A 1975 federal act mandating educational services to all children without exception.

ELECTRODE: An electrical terminal designed for contact with a structure to be stimulated or recorded, as with an EEG.

ELECTROENCEPHALOGRAM (EEG): A recording of the small electrical impulses from cell activity in the cerebral cortex. Useful in identifying areas of cortical damage.

ENCEPHALITIS: An inflammation of the brain resulting from an infection.

ENCEPHALOPATHY: Any disease of the brain.

ENCOPRESIS: Involuntary discharge of the stool.

ENURESIS: Involuntary discharge of urine. With children, usually refers to bedwetting.

ENURETIC SEIZURE: Enuresis associated with seizure, not to be confused with simple nocturnal enuresis.

EPILEPSIA PARTIALIS CONTINUA: Continuous focal-motor seizures.

EPILEPSY: A clinical disorder characterized by recurring attacks of central nervous system dysfunction, which may involve lack of consciousness, convulsive movements, and disturbances of feeling or behavior that are self-limiting.

EPILEPTIC APHASIA: A speech arrest caused by epileptic discharge in regions of the dominant hemisphere of the brain.

EPILEPTIC COMA: A state that follows generalized seizures or status epilepticus.

EPILEPTIC CONFUSION: A confused state occurring during or following generalized seizures.

EPILEPTIC DISCHARGE: An abnormal and excessive electrical discharge from cerebral neurons caused by pathological or genetic factors in some persons with epilepsy.

EPILEPTIC EQUIVALENT: A condition in which some of the symptoms of a seizure appear, but which is not a convulsive motor attack.

EPILEPTIC FOCUS. *See* Seizure focus.

EPILEPTIC FUGUE: Ambulatory or gestural movements of an automatic nature, often following a generalized seizure, and frequently prolonged for up to an hour.

EPILEPTIC HALLUCINATIONS: Various perceptions of smell, taste, feeling, etc., following an attack (like the aura that precedes the attack).

EPILEPTIC PSYCHOSIS: Hallucinations of paranoid character sometimes identified with temporal lobe epilepsy, tending most often to occur in persons whose seizures are tapering off or in response to treatment.

EPILEPTIC SUSCEPTIBILITY: Neurological, physiological, psychological, or genetic factors operating in the brain, leading to a predisposition to epilepsy.

EPILEPTOGENIC: A condition in a person which induces seizure activity, for example, brain lesions.

EPILEPTOLOGIST: A neurologist who specializes in the treatment of epilepsy.

ETHOSUXIMIDE (Zarontin): An anticonvulsant drug used primarily for absence seizures.

ETHOTOIN (Peganone): A second-line drug similar to phenytoin, sometimes used for generalized tonic-clonic and focal-onset seizures.

ETIOLOGY: The cause of a disease or condition.

EUPHORIA: Literally, a state of well-being or elation. In psychiatric application, this feeling may be unrealistic, not consistent with the surroundings. Often of psychological origin; also common among toxic states and organic brain disease.

EXTROVERSION: Interest in other people and the environment (the opposite of introversion). Usually referred to as "outgoingness."

FAMILIAL: Pertaining to or characteristic of a given family, presumably inherited.

FAMILIAL EPILEPSY: The occurrence of epilepsy in several close relatives, considered by some authorities to represent a genetic predisposition.

FEBRILE: Relating to or having a fever.

FEBRILE CONVULSION: An attack brought on by a fever, predominantly among infants and young children. If the seizures continue, they often are considered as epileptic, though febrile convulsions as such are not necessarily epileptic.

FETUS: The unborn offspring in the mother's womb from about the third month until birth.

FOCAL-ONSET SEIZURE: A seizure caused by abnormal electrical discharge in one part of the brain, affecting the part of the body controlled by that part of the brain.

FONTANEL: The soft, boneless area in the skull of a young infant.

FREE-FLOATING ANXIETY: Apprehension or fear of most situations. The person is usually unable to explain this perseverative condition.

FRONTAL LOBE: The area of the central cortex serving as the brain's center for complex associations.

FUGUE: A form of dissociation characterized by amnesia or by a literal physical flight from a threatening situation.

GAMMA-AMINOBUTYRIC ACID (GABA): A substance that alters the normal balance of the nerve cells.

GENE: Any of the parts of the chromosomes that transmit hereditary characteristics.

GENE, DOMINANT: A gene that produces an effect in the offspring, regardless of whether it is matched by a like gene in the chromosome of the mate.

GENE, MULTIPLE: A gene whose individual effects are small and combine with others to produce additive effects.

GENE, RECESSIVE: A gene that produces its effect only when matched by a like gene of the other chromosome of the mate.

GENERALIZED EPILEPSY: Seizures that result from a generalized, nonfocal, electrical discharge in the brain.

GENERALIZED TONIC-CLONIC SEIZURE: A major seizure with alternate stiffening and jerking and loss of consciousness; grand mal.

GENETICS: The branch of science concerned with heredity.

GESELL DEVELOPMENTAL SCHEDULES: A scale for assessing the developmental status (rather than intelligence per se) for infants and young children, aged four weeks to six years. Considered more reliable after the age of six months than for the early months of life.

GESTATION: The period of pregnancy.

GIFTED: Refers to mentally superior ability, or to a student in the top 2 percent of students at similar grade or age level.

GINGIVAL HYPERPLASIA: Enlargement of the gums by increased gum tissue, often induced by certain anticonvulsants (for example, Phenytoin).

GLIA: The connective tissue elements in the brain.

GRAND MAL SEIZURE: *See* Generalized tonic-clonic seizure.

GRAY MATTER: The neural substance of the spinal cord and brain composed primarily of cell bodies.

GUSTATORY: Pertaining to the sense of taste.

GYRI: The ridges on the surface of the brain.

HABILITATION: Improvement in the skill and level of adjustment so as to increase the ability to maintain satisfactory employment or adjustment.

HALFWAY HOUSE: A type of foster home or facility caring for small groups, who may be habilitable or employable in a protective setting.

HALSTEAD-REITAN NEUROLOGICAL TEST BATTERY: A series of tests designed to assess cognitive, perceptual, and motor skills in children (over five years old) and adults.

HEAD START PROGRAM: A federally funded school program for disadvantaged school children, 10 percent of whom must be handicapped.

HEMIPARESIS: Weakness of muscles on one side of the body.

HEMIPLEGIA: Paralysis of one side of the body.

HEMISPHERECTOMY: An operation removing a cerebral hemisphere.

HEREDITARY: Passing naturally from parent to offspring through the genes. Though present in the genes, an inherited trait may not always be apparent in the individual.

HOMEOSTASIS: Maintenance of automatic metabolic or psychological processes, optimal for well-being and survival.

HORMONE: Any of the internally secreted compounds, formed in the endocrine organs, that affect the functioning of certain organs or tissues when carried to them by the body fluids.

HUNTINGTON'S DISEASE: A progressive, inherited disorder which usually begins in the middle years of life, involves choreic movements of the face and/or extremities, and ends in mental deterioration.

HYDROCEPHALUS: An accumulation of cerebrospinal fluid in the cranium often causing an enlargement of the head in infancy and resulting in mental retardation if not arrested early.

HYPERACTIVITY: Uncontrollable, excessive activity.

HYPERSENSITIVITY: Abnormal sensitivity to persons, situations, or other stimuli.

HYPERTHYROIDISM: A condition resulting from excessive secretion by the thyroid gland, marked by excitability, but with no necessary impairment of intellectual functioning.

HYPERVENTILATION: Very rapid breathing.

HYPOGLYCEMIA: Reduction of the concentration of glucose in the blood below the normal level.

HYPOTHALAMUS: The area of the brain which plays an important role in emotions, sleep, and other physiological and psychological functions.

HYPOTHYROIDISM: A condition resulting from lack of secretion by the thyroid gland. A cause of cretinism.

HYPSARRHYTHMIA: A characteristic EEG pattern seen in myoclonic epilepsy in children.

HYSTERICAL SEIZURE: An attack resembling a seizure but not associated with an abnormal discharge in the brain. It is usually psychological in origin. Eighty percent of hysterical seizures occur in patients who also have real seizures.

HYSTERO-EPILEPSY: An older term used to refer to hysterical seizures. Pseudo-epilepsy is another, similar older term.

ICTAL: Pertaining to a seizure.

IDIOGLOSSIA: A condition (other than delayed speech) in which the child's speech is not readily understood.

IDIOPATHIC: Refers to any pathological condition of unknown origin.

IEP: An individual education program, a comprehensive plan developed for a child with special learning problems by a team of professionals.

IMPULSION: A chronic compulsive urge to commit unlawful or disapproved acts.

INFANTILE EPILEPSY: Seizures in the newborn and infants, believed caused by factors such as a predisposition, incomplete cerebral maturation, etc. Seizures are of several types.

INFANTILE MYOCLONIC SEIZURES: Massive seizures in infants, with spasms (salaams), unconsciousness, and autonomic movements. Believed caused by brain malfunction of unknown origin.

INFANT SPASM: A seizure disorder usually occurring during the first year of life and characterized by tonic seizures.

INTEGRATION: The organization of new and old data, emotions, etc., into the personality.

INTELLIGENCE QUOTIENT (IQ): A numerical value assigned to an individual as a result of intelligence testing, with 90–110 being considered the "average" range.

INTERICTAL: Referring to activity between seizures.

INTERICTAL BEHAVIOR: The moods, neuroses, fears, etc., associated with the person's awareness of his condition between seizures.

INTRACRANIAL: Within the skull.

INTROVERSION: Preoccupation with one's self, thus reducing interest in the environment (the opposite of extroversion).

JACKSONIAN SEIZURE: A specialized focal seizure, beginning in the extremities. Not usually generalized, and sometimes can be surgically corrected.

JAUNDICE: Bile pigment in the blood causing the skin to have a yellowish color.

KINDLING: The process of having a seizure induced through repeated electrical stimulation of the brain; done experimentally in animals.

KERNICTERUS: A condition of severe neural symptoms, associated with excessive bilirubin in the blood.

KETOGENIC DIET: A special high-fat, low-carbohydrate diet.

LABILE: Unstable; often refers to vacillating emotions.

LESION: A change in tissue caused by injury or disease.

LIGHTNING SEIZURES: A name given to some infantile myoclonic convulsions because of their rapid appearance and disappearance.

LEARNING PLATEAU: A leveling-off period in the learning process during which no apparent growth is noted.

LENNOX-GASTAUT-WEST SYNDROME: An atypical absence-seizure disorder, with a characteristic EEG pattern.

LOBECTOMY: Excision of a lobe in the brain.

LOBOTOMY: The treatment of serious psychiatric disorders by brain surgery (psychosurgery) in which certain brain nerve fibers are cut to reduce tension and stress.

LOCALIZED: Restricted to a known and limited area.

LOGORRHEA: Compulsive, excessive talking.

MACROCEPHALY: A pathological condition in which the head is especially large and long. Often results in mental retardation.

MEBARAL. *See* Mephobarbital.

MEDULLA: The lower part of the brain above the spinal cord and in front of the cerebellum, which helps regulate heartbeat, blood pressure, and breathing.

MEGAVITAMIN THERAPY: Vitamins given in massive doses.

MENINGITIS: Inflammation of the membranes of the brain or spinal cord, for which no vaccine has yet been found. Considered a frequent cause of epilepsy.

MENTAL AGE (MA): Level of intellectual functioning expressed in terms of years and months, and a basis for determining the IQ.

MENTAL RETARDATION: Mental functioning significantly below the normal. Usually defined in terms of an IQ below 70, with deficient social functioning. Mild retardation refers to those persons who are capable of some degree of achievement in reading, arithmetic, and so on, with IQ scores between 55 and 69. The moderately retarded, with IQ scores between 40 and 54, can be trained to care for their personal needs and work in a sheltered workshop situation. The severely retarded, with IQ range between 25 and 39, require care and rarely become proficient in self-care. Profoundly retarded refers to those with IQs below 24, who usually require total care.

MEPHENYTOIN (Mesantoin): A second-line drug, similar to phenytoin, for treatment of generalized tonic-clonic and focal-onset seizures.

MEPHOBARBITAL: A barbiturate used as an anticonvulsant (Mebaral).

METABOLISM: The chemical changes in cells by which energy is provided for functions and materials assimilated.

METHSUXIMIDE (Celontin): A second-line drug structurally related to ethosuximide, effective against absence seizures, myoclonic jerks, and atonic seizures.

MOTOR: Pertaining to conscious or unconscious muscular movement.

MOTOR NEURON: A neuron conducting impulses away from the central nervous system toward a muscle.

MOTOR PATTERNING: A sensorimotor approach designed to "program" the brain by means of prescribed physical exercises (called Doman-Delacato).

MULTIPLE SCLEROSIS: A progressive and degenerative disease of the central nervous system, caused by a hardening of the tissues of the brain and/or spinal cord.

MUSICOGENIC EPILEPSY: Partial, temporal lobe seizures induced by one's emotional reaction to certain forms of music. Cases are rare.

MUTISM: Refusal or inability to speak.

MYOCLONIC SEIZURE: A generalized convulsive seizure, usually brief in duration, characterized by a sudden massive jerk of the entire body.

MYSOLINE. *See* Primidone.

NARCOLEPSY: A disorder characterized by profound sleepiness during the day, cataplexy, and, occasionally, hallucinations on waking up from sleep or going to sleep.

NEOLOGISM: A new word, series of words, or expressions used in a different context, not readily understood by others. Also frequently used by the emotionally disturbed or psychotic to express complex meanings related to their own conflicts.

NEONATAL: Referring to the period immediately following birth.

NEONATAL ANOXIA: Shortage of oxygen in body tissue of newborn infants.

NEONATAL ASPHYXIA: Inability of the lungs of newborn infants to receive oxygen.

NERVE IMPULSE: An electrochemical excitation passing along nerve cells.

NEUROLOGICAL DAMAGE: Any impairment of the central nervous system.

NEOPLASM: An abnormal growth, such as a tumor.

NEUROLOGIST: A physician trained in diagnosis and treatment of nervous system disorders.

NEUROLOGY: The study of the brain and nervous system.

NEUROMUSCULAR: Pertaining to the relationship between nerves and muscles.

NEURON: Any cell in the central nervous system with the function of transmitting impulses. Also called nerve cell.

NEUROPSYCHIATRIST: A physician who specializes in nervous or psychiatric disorders related to organic disorders of the nervous system. Literally, one who combines the fields of neurology and psychiatry.

NEUROSIS: An emotional difficulty usually caused by unresolved and subconscious conflicts, resulting in partially impaired thinking and judgment. There are innumerable classifications of neuroses, depending on the particular symptom that predominates. No loss of contact with reality is involved, as in cases of psychosis.

NEUROSURGEON: A physician who specializes in brain surgery.

NUTRITION: The process by which the organism receives and absorbs substances into body tissues.

NYSTAGMUS: An involuntary, jerking movement of the eyes.

OBSTETRICS: The branch of medical science dealing with the assistance and care of women during pregnancy, labor, and birth.

OCCIPITAL LOBE: The area of tbe cerebral cortex located at the back of the brain that is the primary center for vision.

OCULAR: Pertaining to the eye.

OLFACTORY: Pertaining to the sense of smell.

OPERANT CONDITIONING: Reinforcement (reward) of desirable behavior to ensure repetition of the behavior, leading toward a habit pattern.

OPHTHALMOLOGIST: A physician who specializes in eye diseases and their cure.

ORGANIC: Pertaining to the structure of organs as opposed to their function.

ORGANIC INVOLVEMENT: Any structural condition affecting mental, motor, or communicative functions, caused by brain injury (for example, cerebral palsy, epilepsy, etc.).

ORTHODONTIA: The branch of dentistry concerned with the straightening of dental structures, aligning of teeth, and prevention of irregularities.

ORTHOPEDICALLY HANDICAPPED (OH): Any child who, because of physical impairment, cannot receive the full benefit of regular classroom activities and is thus eligible for special class.

OSSIFICATION: The formation of bone.

PALSY: Impairment of motor function because of brain injury.

PARAPLEGIA: Paralysis of the lower half of the body.

PARESIS: Slight or partial motor paralysis.

PARIETAL LOBE: The area of the cerebral hemisphere lying behind the central sulcus and in front of the occipital lobe.

PAROXYSMAL: Referring to a sudden, periodic attack or recurrence of symptoms.

PARTIAL EPILEPSY: Focal, localized epilepsy.

PATHOGNOMONIC: Referring to a group of symptoms related to a disease or condition (similar to syndrome).

PATHOPHYSIOLOGY: The study of abnormal (pathological) functioning of a body part.

PEDIATRICIAN: A physician who specializes in the care of children.

PEGANONE. *See* Ethotoin.

PERCENTILE: A way to express one's ranking in terms of the percentage of the population falling below the person in a given area (for example, to be in the 20th percentile means that out of 100 people, approximately 20 would fall below the person and 80 above him).

PERCEPTION: The process of selecting, organizing, and integrating sensory data.

PERINATAL: The period of life from birth to one week after birth.

PERSEVERATION: Behavior causing a person to continue pursuing a task after the need for it has passed. Often associated with neurological damage.

PETIT MAL SEIZURE. *See* Absence seizure.

PHENOBARBITAL: The oldest and most widely used anticonvulsant.

PHENOTHIAZINE: An important chemical in the transmission of impulses from one nerve fiber to another across a synaptic junction; the basic chemical neuromuscular transmitter to activate the muscles.

PHENYLALANINE: A derivative from protein; an amino acid essential for human metabolism.

PHENYLKETONURIA (PKU): An inability of the body to assimilate phenylalanine, causing irreversible mental retardation unless corrected early.

PHENYTOIN (Dilantin): An anticonvulsant drug for focal-onset, secondarily generalized tonic-clonic, and generalized-onset tonic-clonic seizures.

PHOBIA: An unrealistic fear, often accompanied by compulsive avoidance mechanisms.

PHOTIC STIMULATION: Stimulation by light.

PHOTOGENETIC SEIZURE: A seizure induced by intermittent light stimulation. A common type of reflex seizure, occasionally self-induced by children.

PHOTOPHOBIA: Aversion of or intolerance to light.

PLACENTA: A structure in the uterus through which the fetus receives its nourishment and disposes of its wastes.

PLACEBO: An inactive substance without therapeutic value, which the patient considers "real."

PLACEBO EFFECT: The psychological response of patients who have received a placebo, unaware that it has no therapeutic effect and thinking it has value.

PLAY THERAPY: A therapeutic approach to children's disorders in which the observation and interpretation of the child's use of materials and his fantasy in his games and play form part of the basis for the therapy.

PNEUMOENCEPHALOGRAM: An X-ray picture of the skull and its contents after the injection of air or gas into the brain spaces.

POSTICTAL: Following a seizure.

POST-TRAUMATIC EPILEPSY: Epilepsy following a severe injury to the head.

PRECONSCIOUS: Referring to data or thoughts that are not in the immediate awareness but that can be recalled by conscious effort.

PREICTAL: Preceding a seizure.

PRIMIDONE (Mysoline): An anticonvulsant drug used for generalized tonic-clonic and focal-onset seizures.

PROGNOSIS: Prediction based upon current evidence.

PROJECTIVE TECHNIQUE: A device (test, inventory, interview, etc.) in which the subject is asked to describe, invent, relate, etc., and project himself into the response.

PROPHYLAXIS: Any preventive treatment of disease.

PSEUDO-RETARDATION: A condition exhibited by a person who tests at the level of the retarded but who does not present the picture of any of the clinical categories of retardation. There may be emotional, cultural, academic, or other causes.

PSYCHIATRIST: A physician who specializes in mental disorders.

PSYCHIC SEIZURE: A focal (partial) seizure identified with emotional manifestations, such as hallucinations, affective reactions, etc.

PSYCHOGENIC: Caused by emotional rather than physiological factors.

PSYCHOLOGIST: One trained in the understanding of behavior and its relationship to the environment. A clinical psychologist would be one trained in the diagnosis and treatment of behavioral and mental disorders.

PSYCHOMETRICS: The measurement and evaluation of intelligence and other aspects of behavior, performed by a psychologist or psychiatrist.

PSYCHOMOTOR SEIZURE: A temporal lobe seizure accompanied by automatic motor activity.

PSYCHOSIS: A severe emotional disorder, resulting in loss of contact with reality.

PSYCHOTHERAPY: Group or individual treatment of various psychological disorders by a qualified, trained therapist.

RAPPORT: In counseling, the client-counselor relationship.

READING DISABILITY: Inadequate reading skill, usually two or more grades below the norm.

READING EPILEPSY: A form of seizure believed induced by the rapid eye movements needed in reading, or by the intellectual or emotional reaction to the stimulation while reading.

REFLEX EPILEPSY: Seizures induced by sensory stimulation, for instance, auditory, visual, startle, etc.

REFLEX INHIBITION: The opposite of a reflex seizure, in which the sensory stimulation may inhibit or prevent a seizure.

REGRESSION: The partial (or symbolic) readoption of more infantile means of gratification. The person subconsciously "returns" to a stage in his development in which he felt more secure.

REMISSION: A time period when the symptoms are not present.

REPRESSION: An automatic mechanism by which a person rejects from his conscious level any unbearable thoughts or impulses. Though the thoughts are buried in the subconscious, they may emerge in disguised form, such as, phobias, etc.

RESISTANCE: An individual's psychological defense against bringing repressed thoughts, ideas, fears into his awareness.

RESPITE CARE: Placement or services to provide temporary relief for parents.

RH INCOMPATIBILITY: A problem based on a blood factor identical with one found in the rhesus monkey (hence the name, Rh). When a mother is Rh negative and a father Rh positive, their baby may be mentally retarded or seriously ill. The incompatibility is correctable in early stages.

ROENTGENOGRAPHIC: Pertaining to photography by X ray.

RUBELLA: German measles; when suffered by the pregnant mother, especially during the first trimester, frequently causes mental retardation in the fetus.

RUBEOLA: Hard measles. Immunization now required in school pupils in most states.

SALAAM EPILEPSY: Spasms associated with infantile myoclonic seizures.

SCHOOL PHOBIA: A syndrome in which the pupil resists or refuses to go to school. Symptoms often include tears, nausea, tenseness, or defiance. Causes vary, but are believed often to be related to separation anxiety.

SCOTOMA: A "blind spot" in one's perceptual awareness.

SECONDARY EPILEPSY: Seizures of an acquired type, for example, metabolic, toxic, etc.

SEIZURE: An attack of sudden abnormal electrical discharge in the brain causing transient disturbance of brain function and affecting body systems.

SEIZURE FOCUS: The particular location in the brain of the abnormal electrical discharge.

SELECTIVE PERCEPTION: The tendency to see or hear what we want to see or hear, disregarding other conflicting or contradictory stimuli.

SELF-ACTUALIZATION: The optimal state, in which one accepts himself as functioning at capacity.

SELF-CONCEPT (or self-esteem): One's total opinion of himself, which is believed vitally to affect the level of functioning. This impression is highly influenced by our perception of how others see us.

SELF-INDUCED SEIZURE: A generalized seizure, more commonly found in children, induced deliberately by photic stimulation or by hyperventilation.

SENSORY SEIZURE: A partial (focal) seizure with accompanying sensations, such as hallucinations.

SEQUELA: An after-effect of a disease.

SHELTERED WORKSHOP: A vocational facility in which the handicapped can work in a protective, noncompetitive setting under supervision.

SIBLING: A brother or sister.

SKULL SERIES: X rays of the brain and skull.

SLOW LEARNERS: A term applied to those school children who tend to obtain IQ scores between 75 and 90, who are able to profit from school, but who usually need vocational training after grade eight.

SODIUM VALPROATE. *See* Valproic acid.

SOMATHESTHESIA: Consciousness of body feelings or sensations.

SPASM: Literally, a prolonged muscular contraction, often used to describe a childhood seizure.

SPASTICITY: Tightness of the muscles, causing spasms and an inability to control motor operations.

SPEECH PATHOLOGIST: A speech specialist who discovers, diagnoses, and treats speech disorders.

SPIKE: A term used in electroencephalography to denote a triangular-shaped wave that is sudden in appearance and out of keeping with the background brain-wave activity; less than 80 milliseconds in duration.

SPIKE-AND-SLOW-WAVE DISCHARGE: A brain-wave pattern of spikes and slower inhibitory waves. The hallmark of a seizure focus, it usually appears in between seizures.

SPINAL CORD: The neural structure encased in the backbone that serves as a pathway for impulses to and from the brain.

SPINAL NERVES: The 31 pairs of nerves connected to the spinal cord.

SSI: Supplemental Security Income, a program providing cash benefits for needy persons, including the handicapped.

STANFORD-BINET, L-M: A widely used intelligence test for ages two years through superior adult.

STARTLE SEIZURE: Reflex seizure, generalized, induced by sudden changes or unexpected sensory stimulation.

STATUS EPILEPTICUS: A series of prolonged seizures, with little or no time between seizures, often accompanied by signs of interference with vital functions. Requires immediate medical attention. Usually caused by too rapid a change in medication.

STIGMATA: The characteristics or marks of a given condition.

STIMULUS: Any energy capable of attracting, stimulating, or exciting the nervous system.

STRABISMUS: Inability to direct the eyes to the same point as a result of imbalance in eye muscle control.

STRESS: Any strong emotional tension.

STURGE-WEBER SYNDROME: A congenital syndrome involving vascular changes of the face and eyes, associated with intracranial calcification, mental retardation, and epilepsy.

SUBCLINICAL EPILEPSY: Seizures so mild that they are not easily recognizable; they are detectable mainly by perceptual psychometric testing or by irregular EEG activity.

SUBCORTICAL EPILEPSY: Epilepsy that is believed to originate from neural discharge in the subcortical areas of the brain.

SUBDURAL HEMATOMA: A massive blood clot in the brain.

SUBICTAL STATE: A sudden epileptic symptom without a seizure.

SULCI: The deep fissures, or grooves, in the surface of the brain that separate the ridges, or gyri, and the lobes.

SUTURES: The spaces between the bones of the skull.

SYMPTOM: A behavioral or physiological manifestation or clue to an existing condition.

SYMPTOMATIC: Having a known, identifiable origin.

SYNCOPE: Fainting.

SYNDROME: A group of symptoms that make up a clinical entity.

TACHISTOSCOPE: A device for presenting visual recognition items for extremely brief periods of time. Often used for developing speed in letter, form, or word recognition.

TEGRETOL. *See* Carbamazepine.

TELEMETRY: An EEG recording of a patient, done while the patient is engaged in a variety of normal-life situations. Useful in determining the factors that may bring on seizures.

TEMPORAL LOBE: The area of the cerebral cortex in front of the occipital lobe with centers for hearing, speech, perceptions, and other associations.

TEMPORAL LOBE EPILEPSY: Focal (or partial) seizures originating in or near the temporal lobe, usually preceded by the aura.

THERAPY: Treatment or remedies.

TONIC: Referring to persistent, involuntary muscular contractions.

TONIC SEIZURE: A short generalized seizure in infancy, marked by a period of unconsciousness and autonomic activity.

TOXEMIA: A bacterial condition in which the blood contains toxic or poisonous substances.

TRAUMA: Any severe emotional shock or injury.

TREMOR: An involuntary shaking or muscular movement of the body, most often involving the head or limbs.

TRIMESTER, FIRST: The first three months of pregnancy.

TUBEROUS SCLEROSIS: Hardening of the tissues of the brain by tumors and often characterized by mental deterioration and seizures. Considered familial.

TUMOR: An abnormal swelling or tissue growth.

UNCINATE SEIZURE: A type of temporal lobe, focal epilepsy, often associated with olfactory symptoms and/or hallucinations.

UNDERACHIEVEMENT: Achievement (usually meant to be academic) markedly below one's evidenced potential, as opposed to low achievement, in which one merely performs at a low level of competence.

UNDIFFERENTIATED: Referring to causes that are unknown. Used frequently with reference to certain forms of mental retardation.

UNILATERAL SEIZURE: A focal seizure involving only one side of the body.

VALIDITY: The extent to which a given test, technique, etc., does what it purports to do.

VALIUM. *See* Diazepam.

VALPROIC ACID (sodium valproate, Depakene): A new anticonvulsant used mainly for petit-mal absence seizures.

VENTRICLES: The communicating cavities in the brain that are continuous with the central canal of the spinal cord.

VINELAND SCALE OF SOCIAL MATURITY: A test that measures the social development of persons of all ages, occasionally scored with the aid of a parent or other informant. The score is reported as a social age (SA) or social quotient (SQ).

WECHSLER INTELLIGENCE SCALES: A group of intelligence tests measuring verbal and performance abilities for children from age three through age sixteen and adults.

WIDE RANGE ACHIEVEMENT TEST (WRAT): An individual academic achievement test for virtually any grade level, including nursery school, that gives grade-level equivalent scores in spelling, reading, and arithmetic.

WORKSHOP, SHELTERED. *See* Sheltered Workshop.

ZARONTIN. *See* Ethosuximide.

INDEX

Absence seizures (petit mal), 8, 10, 11,
12, 17, 18, 19, 32, 39, 43, 44, 45,
49, 73, 138, 170, 182
characteristics of, 15–16, 65
medication for, 88, 89, 90, 91–92
Absence variant, 15
Acceptance, 129
Accidents, 35, 68–69
Acetazolamide (Diamox), 52, 89–90
ACTH. *See* Corticotropin
Adolescents, 68, 94, 111, 125, 126,
132–133, 150–151, 161, 172
Adoption, 186
Adult adjustments, 35–36, 134–135
Age:
and disability benefits, 156
and hyperactivity, 51
and insurance, 172, 177
and knowledge of disease, 115–116
and Medicare, 178
and mortality, 178–179
and motor devlopment, 21, 22
and myoclonic seizures, 17
and pregnancy, 51
and prevalency of epilepsy, 43–44,
47
and prognosis, 44, 46
and seizure onset, 18–19, 30, 32
and self-esteem, 111

and special education, 145, 149,
152, 153
and speech, 22–24, 114
and treatment, 67, 84
Akinetic seizures, 8, 11, 17, 49
Alcohol, 1, 30, 33, 38, 52, 79–80, 169,
182, 184
Alexander the Great, 3
Allergy, 92
American Epilepsy Society, 61, 62
American Medical Association, 185
Amphetamines, 90
Anemia, 51
Angel Unaware (Evans and Rogers),
131–132
Anger, 128–129, 132
Annegers, J., 45
Anticonvulsants, 178, 184, 192
adjustments in, 44, 67–68
and alcohol, 79
availability of, 95
and biofeedback, 76–77
and child development, 21, 102
cost of, 82, 83, 98–99
and driving, 182, 197–202
and drug addiction, 98
and febrile convulsions, 14
and fetal abnormalities, 52–53
forms of, 97–98

Anticonvulsants *(cont.)*
  guidelines, 84–85, 96–97
  and hyperactivity, 50
  and inequities in financial assistance
    for, 188–189
  and insurance, 168
  and ketogenic diet, 77, 78
  and mental retardation, 48
  and military service, 187
  obtaining through EFA, 99, 165
  and post-traumatic seizures, 35
  and pregnancy, 51, 52–53
  purposeful failure to take, 38, 132
  and remission, 45, 46, 79
  resistance to, of myoclonic seizures,
    17
  at school, 141
  specific drugs, 85–92
  and status epilepticus, 18, 75, 90, 95
  and surgery qualifications, 70, 71
  timing of, 94–96, 97, 105, 132
  See also Side effects; *specific drugs*
Anxiety, 122, 128, 131
Aphasia, 148
Aplastic anemia, 86–87, 89
Arteriovenous malformations
  (AVMs), 19, 65, 66
Arteriogram, 60
"Assigned risk," 176
Ataxia, 89, 90, 92, 93
Atonic seizures, 8, 11, 13, 17, 88, 89,
  90
Attwell, A., 21
Atypical petit mal, 15, 47
Audiovisual aids, 62
Aura, 12, 77
Autism, 152
Automobile insurance, 170, 176
Autonomic epilepsy, 16
Autry, James, 197

Baby-sitter, 134, 164
Bagley, C., 25
Bahler, W., 76
Balance problems, 24, 87, 88, 90, 93
Bankers Life and Casualty Insurance,
  169
Barbiturates, 30
Battered children, 34

Bayley Scales of Infant Development,
  61
Bear, D. M., 27
Because You Are My Friend, 126
Bed-wetting, 119
Behavior disorders, 49, 51, 88, 103,
  108, 142, 154
Behavior modification, 77
Benjamin, 126
Berger, Hans, 62
Bilateral massive epileptic myoclonus,
  8, 11
Biofeedback, 76–77
Birth injury, 29, 30–31, 34, 50, 68
Birth order, 34
Blood tests, 59, 61, 68, 84–85, 87, 88,
  93, 115
"Bona fide occupational qualifica-
  tions" (BFOQ), 192
Bone marrow, 86, 89, 92
Books, 125–126, 131–132
Brain:
  and causes of epilepsy, 29–31, 34
  cell metabolism, 71
  and diagnostic tests, 59–60, 62–67
  functions and areas of, 3–7
  injury to, 16, 29, 35–36, 44, 47, 48,
    70
  and learning disabilities, 143
  and mental illness, 26, 27
  and seizures, 2, 8–9, 12, 17, 18, 24,
    47–48
  and status epilepticus, 75
  and strokes, 19
  surgery, 69–71, 79
Brain encephalopathy, 17
Brain tumors, 29, 30, 65–66
Brain waves, 7, 15–16, 63, 76, 90–91.
  See also Electroencephalogram
Breath–holding, 20
Breger, E., 133
British Epilepsy Association, Medical
  Advisory Committee, 182
Bruising, 88
Buddha, 3

Caesar, Julius, 3
Calculus (tartar), 94
Camp, 118–119, 165

Pity, 119–120, 128
Platelets, blood, 88
Pneumoencephalogram, 60, 67, 70
Post-traumatic seizures, 16, 35–36, 69
Power tools, 138
Pregnancy, 33, 51, 52–53, 68–69, 127
Premature birth, 47
Prenatal care, 68
Prevalency of epilepsy, 40–42, 43–47, 53–54
Prevention of epilepsy, 35, 68–69
Primidone (Mysoline), 52, 86, 87–88, 90, 91
Prisoners, 25, 26
Prognosis for epilepsy, 18–19, 45–46
Projects With Industry (PWI), 194
Prudential Insurance Company, 169
Pseudoseizure, 17
Psychiatric illnesses, 26, 27
Psychological problems, 26, 35–36, 67, 108, 183. *See also* Emotional problems
Psychological examinations, 60–61, 67, 70
Psychologist. *See* Clinical psychologist
Psychomotor epilepsy, 9, 12, 26, 32–33, 49, 86, 138, 184, 186. *See also* Partial seizures with complex symptomatology
Psychoses. *See* Psychiatric illnesses
PTA, 130
Public opinion and knowledge, 107, 108–109, 110, 122, 123, 183, 189–190
Pyridoxine deficiency, 30

Quaaludes, 30

Radioactive-labeled glucose, 71
Reading:
  and learning problems, 143
  seizures induced by, 37
Records, seizure, 104
Reflex epilepsy, 36–37, 38
Rehabilitation Act (1973), 159, 190–191, 192
Religious view, 121, 131–132
Remission, 44, 45–46, 79
Research:

costs, 83
need for, 39, 53, 68, 196
support for, 124, 165–166
Residential placement. *See* Housing
Respiratory seizures, 16
Ridicule, 107
Ritalin, 50
Role of the School Nurse in the Understanding and Treatment of Epilepsy, The, 140
Rose, S. W., 40, 41
Run, Patty, Run (Cragg), 55

Seat belts, 35, 69
Schizophrenia, 26
School:
  and academic success, 151
  difficulties at, 142–143
  education of personnel, 140–141
  environment, 136–139
  informing about child's epilepsy. 136–137
  and laws, 145, 146, 148, 149
  medication at, 141
  and special classes, 142
  and vocational education, 150–151
  See also Education; Teacher
School bus, 148–149
School nurse, 136, 141
Sedation. *See* Sleep
Seizure discharge. *See* Electrical discharge
Seizure focus, 7, 19, 70–71
Self-esteem, 110–111, 128, 132, 133, 147
Self-help groups, 125, 130
Self-induced seizures, 37–38, 104
Self-relaxing techniques, 120
Sensory area, 6, 19
Serum level of medications, 85, 93
Sex differences and hyperactivity, 50–51
Sexuality:
  and parental adjustment, 129
  and seizures, 25
Sexual seizures, 16
Sheltered workshop, 162–163
Siblings, 15, 32, 102, 103, 104, 116–118
Side effects:

Side effects (*cont.*)
of carbamazepine, 86–87
of clonazepam, 90
of dextroamphetamine, 90
and driving, 182
of ethosuximide, 89
of ethotoin, 89
importance of, 84, 85, 91, 92–93, 96
of mephenytoin, 89
of methsuximide, 90
of phenobarbital, 87
of phenytoin, 87, 94
of primidone, 88
and sluggishness, 93–94
of valproic acid, 88
Skill areas, 147, 149
Skin rash, 92
Sleep, 11, 182
deprivation, 1, 38, 60
seizures during, 74, 106
as side effect, 89, 90, 93, 96
See also Drowsiness
Sluggishness, 93–94
Smoking, 33, 52
Social development, 60–61, 147, 152, 189, 196
Social Security Act, Title XX, 155, 158
Social Security Administration, 155, 156–157
Social Security Disability Insurance, 177, 188–189
Social worker, 61, 65
Socrates, 3
Sodium-potassium pump, 7
Special education, 83, 124, 130, 142, 143, 144–148, 165
state offices, 239–243
Speech development, 22–24, 60–61, 70, 114–115
Speech therapist, 148, 165
Speed limit, 35, 69
Spike-and-slow-wave discharge, 7, 15, 65, 70, 90–91
Spinal fluid, 65
Stanford-Binet Intelligence Scale, 61
States:
and driver's licensing, 180–182, 197–202
and federal laws and programs, 153–154, 155, 157, 159–160

Status epilepticus, 18, 75, 76, 90, 95, 197
Stealing, 112–113
Sterilization, 186
Sterman, Barry, 76
Stress, 1, 2, 31, 38, 39, 69, 96, 112, 120, 164
Strokes, 19, 29, 30, 65
Sturge-Weber's disease, 57
Stuttering, 148
"Substandard" insurance groups, 171–172, 173
Suicide, 26
Sulci, 4
Supplemental Security Income (SSI), 155–157, 187–188
Surgery, 69–72, 79
Suzuki study, 91
Swimming, 106, 138
Symptoms:
of potential epilepsy, 137
reporting unusual, 96

"Tactile" epilepsy, 36–37
Tchaikovsky, P. I., 3
Teachers, 49, 107, 111, 150
education of, 136–137, 139–140
and laws, 146
and precautions, 137–138
and potential seizure symptoms, 137
reaction to seizures, 138–139
and School Alert program, 140–141
See also Education; School
Teacher's Tips About the Epilepsies, 140
Teach Your Child to Talk, 115
Teenagers. *See* Adolescents
Tegretol. *See* Carbamazepine
Temporal lobe, 3, 4
Temporal lobe epilepsy, 9, 86, 91, 186, 189
and birth order, 34
and learning disabilities, 143
and psychosis, 26, 27
and sexuality, 25
and suicides, 26
and surgery, 69–70
Therapeutic range of medications, 85, 86, 88, 91, 93
Thrombosis, 19